Healthy Weight, Healthy You!

Achieving your ideal weight by exploring the mind-body connection to weight loss.

Charlene Marie Muhammad

First published by Dog Ear Publishing
4010 W. 86th Street, Ste H
Indianapolis, IN 46268
www.dogearpublishing.net

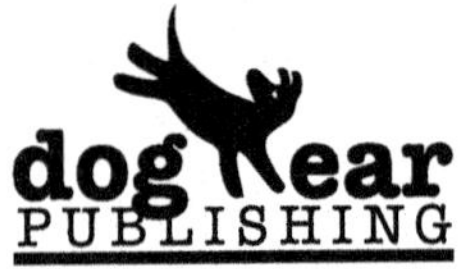

ISBN: 978-1-4575-2982-5

Library of Congress Control Number: has been applied for

This book is printed on acid-free paper.

Printed in the United States of America

Sections:

I. The mind-body connection to food 3

II. Brief History of the American Diet 11

III. Your two brains 16

IV. Tools to increase our awareness for eating healthier 20

V. What's the best diet on the market today? 28

VI. Simple steps for a healthier lifestyle 33

VII. Kitchen Science Wisdom 36

VIII. Exercise Mood & Food 41

Resources

- FAQs
- Supplement materials (handouts)
- Sample menus
- Additional resources by section
- Bibliography

Acknowledgements

The only original thought IS THE original thought (I believe it goes something like this: *In the beginning was the Word…*), therefore it is my honor to thank all who shared their thoughts, reflections, criticisms and time to this project.

Huge gratitude to Cindi Miller and her staff at John Hopkins Medicine's Howard County General Hospital Wellness Center for providing me with a venue to share my passion and knowledge of health and wellness with the community. Thanks also to all those who participated in the quarterly Healthy Weight Loss series over the past three years, for it is you who have taught me much about the human quest for wellness. Much appreciation to Efua Morgan, the first pair of eyes I cautiously beseeched to read my manuscript and who fed me positive advice and editorial guidance.

Humble gratitude to the best family clan and inner circle of friends who feed my spirit everyday- I am in awe by your strength and perseverance!

And a deep bow of gratitude to the Creator and Sustainer of Life. My heart rejoices for I know I am nestled in Your Bosom. I pray my life is a testimony of service for all that is Good.

Salaam. Namaste. Peace.

INTRODUCTION

Greetings!

Healthy Weight, Healthy You! is a companion guide to a healthy weight loss workshop series developed by me. After years of conducting these workshops, writing handouts and recipes and then making multiple copies for participants, I was lucky enough to entertain an idea- given to me by one of the workshop participants- to package all of the information into one convenient volume. Hopefully, this will also save some trees.

The *Healthy Weight, Healthy You!* workshop series was created to help folks like you, kick-start individual lifestyle changes. I am striving to provide a well-rounded; "holistic" approach to achieving weight loss goals. One truth I know for sure, there is no magic bullet to weight loss. It takes time, patience and discipline. However, the more you know and understand about yourself- how you feel, think and act- the better you are:

- taking your time with the process because you begin to enjoy learning about yourself in new ways;
- developing the patience to support your own strengths and challenges; and
- creating a discipline that keeps you going consistently every day.

The *Healthy Weight, Healthy You!* workbook is also designed as a self-study guide. I refer to a variety of research, books and other resources throughout the workbook that will lead you to dig deeper in the study of the topic that is reference. Be sure to read the end-notes and bibliography.

Enjoy!

They who look upon food as the Lord's Gift shall never lack life's physical comforts.
From food are made all bodies.
All bodies feed on food and it feeds on all bodies.

~Taittiriya Upanishad (vs. 142)

I.

THE MIND-BODY CONNECTION TO FOOD

The gift of life is health. Health is actively living as nature intended. It is understanding our purpose in creation and fulfilling that purpose to the best of our ability.
What does it mean to live as nature intended? How do we begin to understand our purpose for being on the planet?

The Wellness Continuum

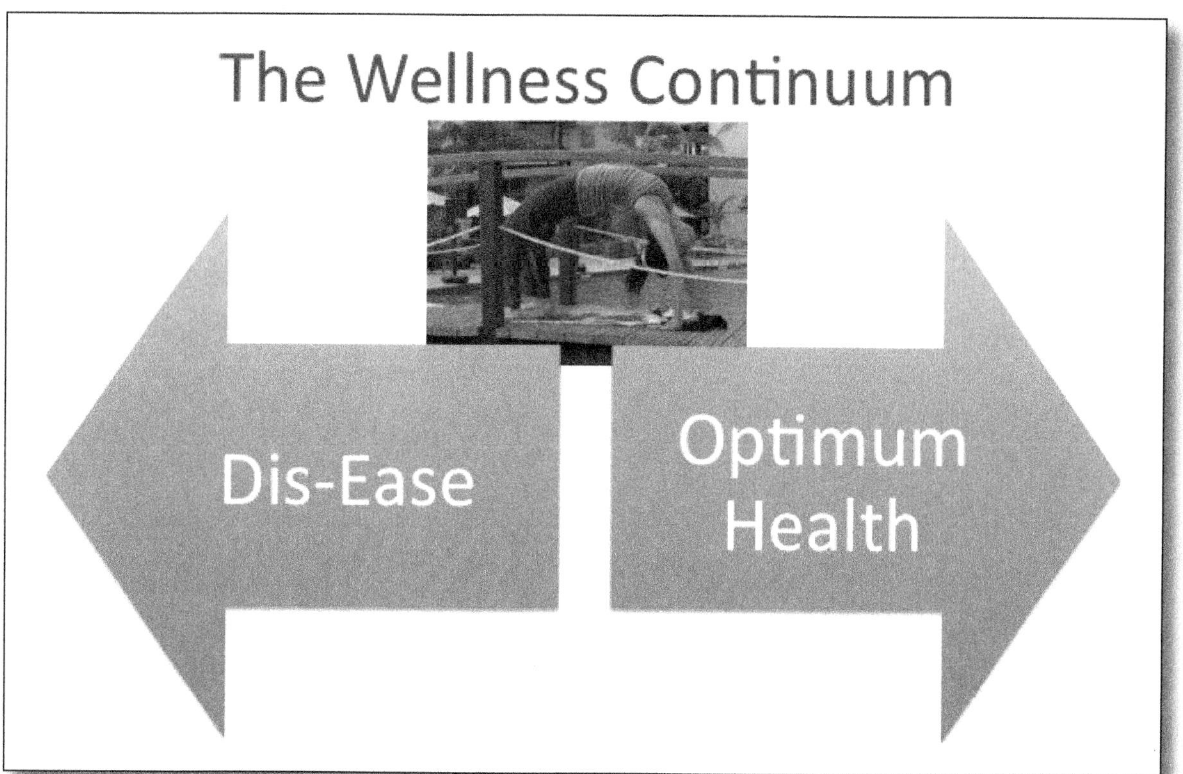

I am honored to borrow this particular concept of a Wellness Continuum from one of our health pioneer's, Dr. John Chissell, who lived and worked in Baltimore, Maryland at Johns Hopkins Hospital. He wrote a book called *Pyramids of Power! An Ancient African Centered Approach to Optimal Health*[1] that explores the mind-body-spirit connections to health and disease.

The Wellness Continuum observes life as fluid- always moving and never stagnant. I like to think of life as a spiral, constantly moving upward. However, at times, we can get stuck in a pattern that feels like we are moving in circles rather than advancing forward like spirals. During these life episodes, we should pay especially close attention because great lessons are learned in these seemingly circular places. With lessons learned, we move more quickly up the spiral towards "higher ground" as Stevie Wonder would say[2] or to wiser outlooks on life.

In other words, your personal wellness flows along a continuum ever oscillating between feeling good and feeling not so good or as Dr. Chissell noted in his book between feeling and being "at" ease or feeling and being in "dis" ease.

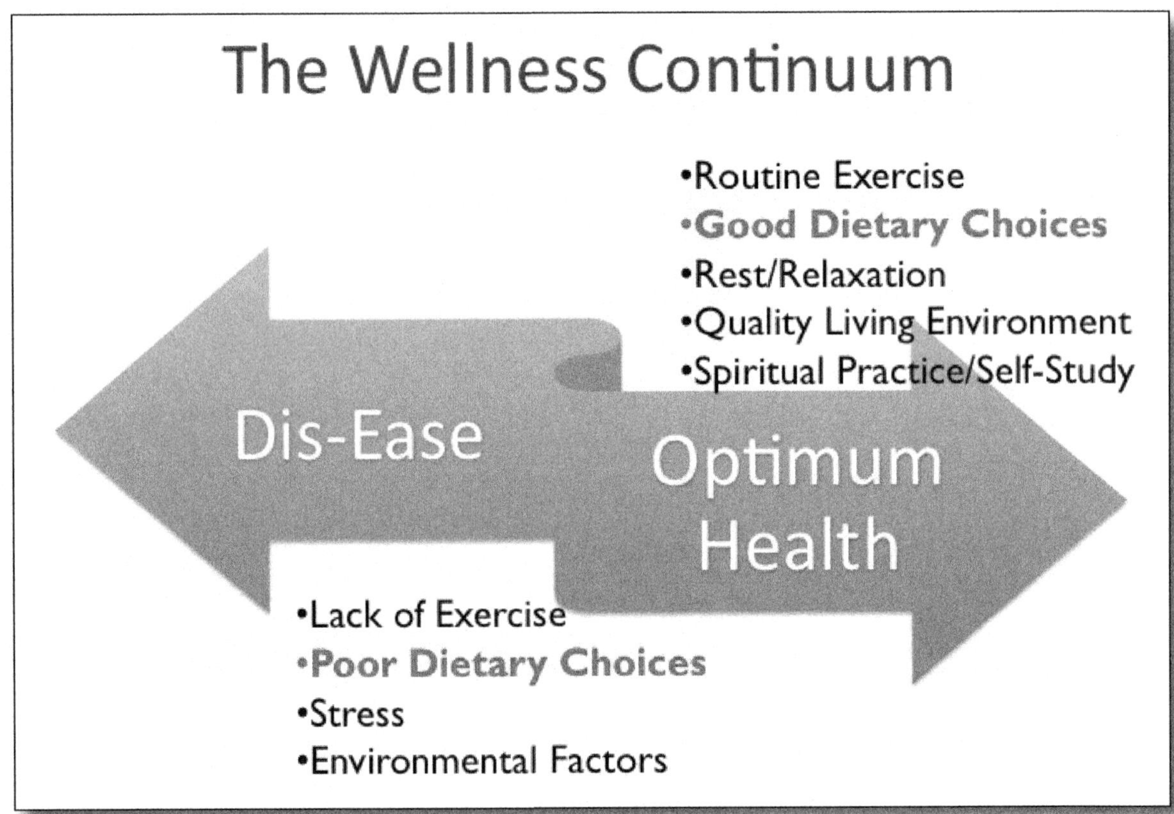

> *"...The concept of health promotion and disease prevention means that we start doing, and continue doing, those things that move use toward optimal health and stop doing those things that move us toward disease and premature death.*[3]

There are many factors or ingredients that make up the wellness continuum: factors that impact your movement through life that leads you towards dis-ease or more towards optimal health. Some of these factors are:

- Exercise or the lack of exercise
- The quality of the environment you live in
- Life style choices: rest, relaxation or stress; spiritual practice (self- study) or workaholic syndrome
- Diet choices: the foods that you eat and/or choose not to eat

Notice how the same factors- depending on the choices you make- can lead you toward dis-ease or towards optimal health. Why is this? Because as human beings, we are a part of nature, interconnected, influenced and impacted by all of the forces in the universe: natural and man-made.

> *The human is a willful, vibrant, idiosyncratic wonderful being, not to be divided into compartments, whether these are of "body", "mind" and "spirit", or separate functional fragments; all living beings are inherently self-regulating, and in health their functions are totally integrated and barely identifiable; disorders, however, manifest as patterns of dysfunction that can be recognized, charted and interpreted to the benefit of any healing intervention.*[4]

Of these many factors, diet appears to impact us the most: physically, mentally and emotionally.

The Power of Food

Remember the classic Dickens' tale, *Oliver Twist*? Oliver's troubles began because he asked for a piece of bread. It was all down hill from there.

Food, glorious food!
What wouldn't we give for?
That extra bite more—
That's all we live for!"[5]

Why do we wish and live for food?
What is food and what is its purpose in our lives?

Food is the Staff of Life

Nature provides us with sources of "life" to sustain our "lives".
We call this food- or as the American Heritage Dictionary defines it: *any material, usually of plant or animal origin, containing or consisting of essential body nutrients…that is taken in and assimilated by an organism to maintain life and growth.*[6]

Food aids nature's gift of health. The life giving sources of food are its nutrients or chemical compounds. This nourishment integrates with human biochemistry and the union between nutrients and biochemistry affects every organ system within your body ultimately leading to optimal health or disease.

70% of the food in today's typical diet that we eat here in the west was virtually unknown to our ancestors.[7] These include:

Cereals, rice and pastas
Dairy products
Added salt
Refined vegetable oils
Refined sugars
Fatty meats

Refined sugars, grains, vegetable oils and diary products make up 70.9% of the energy (what keeps us alive, awake and moving) in the United States food supply, supplanting the whole foods and minimally processed food sources of our ancestors.[8]

Why does this matter?

Because this basic CHANGE in our food supply has made us move to the left of the wellness continuum: towards a lifestyle of DIS- EASE.

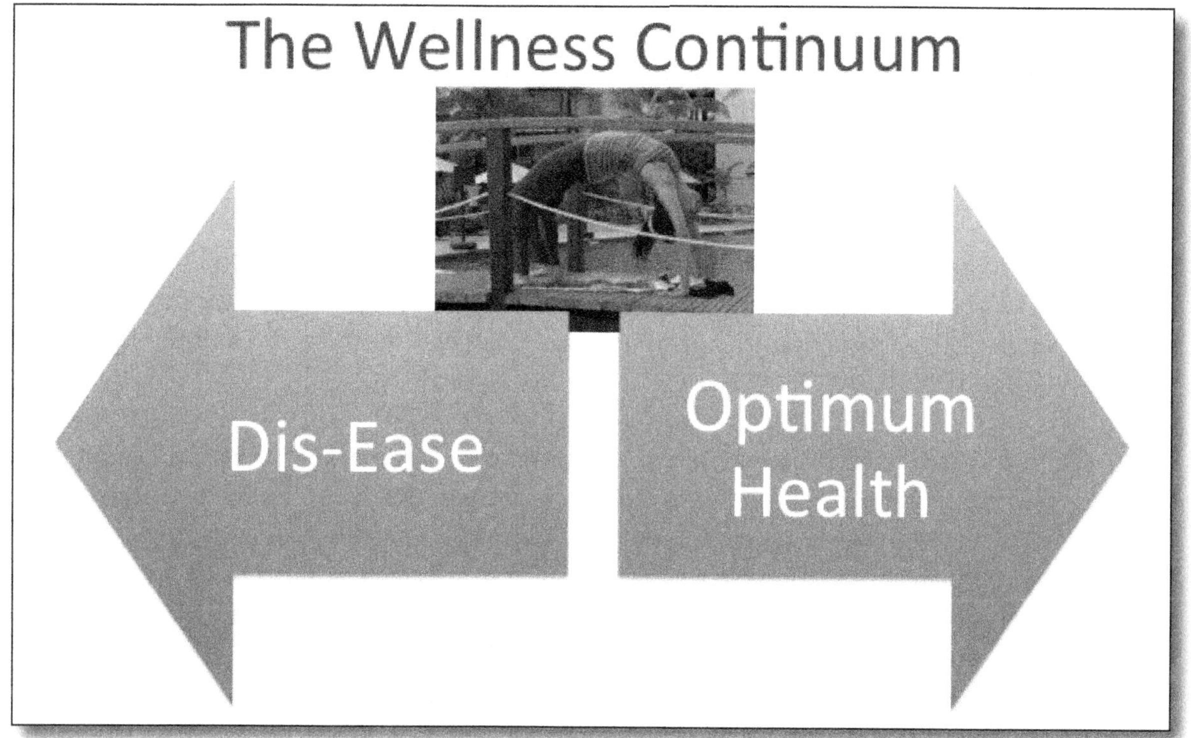

The Unfavorable Effects of the Western Diet

Because we no longer eat food sources that are closest to their natural state when grown and produced, we do not receive the vital nutrients (vitamins, minerals, good fat, fiber and protein) that we need to maintain our health.
The lost of these nutrients are the underlying cause for much of the chronic diseases in the world today.

Even though we tend to over-eat, we are nutrient deficient. Most Americans don't eat the recommended daily allowance (RDA) for one or more essential nutrient on a daily basis.[9]

Most Americans don't eat the United States Department of Agriculture's (USDA) suggested 3 servings of vegetables or 2 servings of fruit daily.[10] This recommendation is based on research that shows eating these servings will provide you with the ***minimum*** amount of nutrients you need to maintain good health.

What are some of the health risks and physical impacts associated with our typical western diet and lifestyle?[11]

Blood Sugar Imbalance. Sugar or glucose is a source of energy for your body, especially your brain. Your bodies does need sugar, however too much is not good for your health. The glycemic load is the maximum amount of glucose in the blood that needs to be synthesized by the hormone insulin. Imbalances in the glycemic load can interfere with insulin's ability to do its job: too much insulin production or not enough of it can lead to diabetes.

Not Enough Essential Fatty Acids. Essential Fatty Acids (EFAs) like Omega 3, 6 and 9 are "essential" because although you need them, your body cannot produce them. EFAs provide support to several systems of your body- especially the cardiovascular and central nervous systems.

There are two basic types of fat: saturated and unsaturated. **Saturated fats** are fats that are primarily solid in form and come from animals and animal products like milk, cheese, butter and yogurt. The two types of **unsaturated fats**, poly and mono, are primarily liquid in form and come from plant based foods like olives, corn, soy, almonds, and coconut. Unsaturated fats are mainly good sources of EFAs nutrients that our bodies' need for optimal health.

Foods labeled as "Low fat" are made with processed ingredients that are stripped of all or most of its natural fats – good and not so good- can also interfere with healthy body systems. EFAs support cellular integrity or the structure of cells, because your cells' outer membrane is made of fatty tissue. EFAs also decrease the inflammatory response in your body by supporting proper immune function.

Lack of Macronutrients. Macronutrients- proteins, carbohydrates and fats- are vital energy requirements to sustain your health. They support all of the major organ systems of your body.

Proteins are foods that contain complex molecules including amino acids. Proteins provide vital structure and functions to most organ systems, and support the repair of cellular tissue. All meats contain proteins: legumes (beans) eggs and dairy products too.

Carbohydrates are foods that contain lots of sugars or foods that breakdown into sugars during the process of digestion. Carbohydrates can be simple or complex, depending on the molecular structure of the sugars. Whole grains, vegetables and fresh fruits are good sources of carbohydrates because they also contain additional vitamins, minerals and fiber you need. Refined grain products like cake, cookies, breads and pastas are not so good sources of carbohydrates because they lack other nutrients that support optimal health.

As we discussed earlier, **Fats** are lipids and come in both solid (saturated) and liquid (unsaturated) forms, and are "essential" for proper functioning of your body.[12] Fats provide "storage" for your body in the form of adipose tissue, insulating you from the cold and also acting as a reserve for energy when your body has used up all of the calories from carbohydrates. Fat supports healthy skin and hair and also helps you absorb fat-soluble vitamins like Vitamin A, D, E and K.[13]

Most Americans experience an imbalance in macronutrients by either consuming too many fat-rich proteins and carbohydrates that provides twice the amount of calories we need, or on the flip side, attempt to control calorie intake by eating processed low-fat foods that lack the protein and high quality EFAs we need to support cellular membrane integrity.

Limited food intake that are nutrient dense. According to the USDA, Nutrient Dense foods is defined as:

> *...Foods and beverages [that] provide vitamins, minerals, and other substances that may have positive health effects with relatively few calories. The term "nutrient dense" indicates that the nutrients and other beneficial substances in a food have not been "diluted" by the addition of calories from added solid fats, added sugars, or added refined starches, or by the solid fats naturally present in the food. Nutrient-dense foods and beverages are lean or low in solid fats, and minimize or exclude added solid fats, sugars, starches, and sodium. Ideally, they also are in forms that retain naturally occurring components, such as dietary fiber.* [14]

Good, quality micronutrients like vitamins and minerals in the foods you consume, are negatively impacted because they are often stripped from whole foods during processing and then "added" back as synthetic additives. Processing foods like this disrupts the delicate balance of vitamin and minerals that whole foods intuitively provide you in their own natural makeup.

pH imbalance. Acid-base balance is your body's ability to maintain a metabolic neutral state (known as pH) that keeps your body fluids from becoming too acidic (having too much acid) or too basic (having too much alkaline). The pH of water is considered the "standard" because it maintains the most neutral of all substances with a pH of 7. Eating refined or processed foods tend to cause your metabolism to be more acidic than alkaline increasing the inflammatory response in your body. When organ systems are inflamed over a period of time, they begin to wear down. This can lead to other diseases like Leaky Gut Syndrome, Osteoarthritis and Gout.

Sodium/potassium imbalance. Sodium and potassium are two minerals that act as a team. Together, they help regulate the transfer of nutrients and waste products into and outside your cells. Their balance is critical for healthy cells- and healthy bodies! A third of all energy in your body is devoted to maintaining their balance. When there is potassium and sodium balance, cells, nerves and muscles can all function smoothly. Any imbalance in this team's structure- which is almost always due to both an excess of sodium, and a deficiency of potassium- can lead to high blood pressure and unnecessary strain on blood vessels, the heart, and kidneys. Research has shown that there is a direct link between chronic levels of low potassium and kidney disease, lung disorders, hypertension, and stroke. [15]

Lack of Fiber. The "broom" of your gut, fiber supports optimal digestive function. Many foods contain fiber, especially vegetables like celery, dark, green leafies (bok choy, collards and kale); and roots (carrots and yams). Fruits like apples, pears, plums and bananas are also good sources of fiber, as well as whole grains like oats, quinoa and millet. Refine carbohydrates like processed breads, cake, cookies and chips decreased quality fiber in your diet and disrupt digestive function.

The trials of history:
We have been partially held hostage to the Western Diet because it supports the fast paced lifestyle that we choose to live.

If we work 8, 10, 12, 14 hours per day- not including commute time, then what time do we have to prepare sustenance for our families and ourselves?
Fast food was invented to assist us in keeping up with this lifestyle pace; however habitually dining on it is making us SICK!

And this sickness begins with the appearance of excessive WEIGHT GAIN.

- Approximately one in three children are overweight or obese.
- Approximately 68% of American adults (20 years and older) are overweight or obese.

The $17 billion dollar (that's the amount of money the food industry spends marketing to children[16]) questions are:
WHY is this so?
And-
Do we have any CONTROL in this process?

REFLECTION QUESTION

Are your current dietary habits affecting your health? How so?

II.

BRIEF HISTORY OF THE AMERICAN DIET

From agrarian society to industrial society

> *Humans have made three major transitions in the way we secure our food. First we employed hunting and gathering techniques. Then we invented agriculture and produced our food by domesticating plants and animals using human and animal energy inputs to drive the system… In the 1930s we introduced a third era..the 'neocaloric era'..[that] depends almost entirely on imported caloric inputs-fertilizer, pesticides, antibiotics, growth hormones, feed additives, diesel fuel…We continue to use these 'old calories'-…calories that nature has stored for billions of years-at a rapid rate, and since they are 'old calories' they are not renewable.*[17]

The industrial revolution did bring us the ease we so wanted, however it also launched the *couch potato* generation.

The first known use of the phrase *couch potato* was coined in 1982.
Merriam –Webster Dictionary defines "couch potato" as *a lazy and inactive person; especially one who spends a great deal of time watching television.* [18]
Merriam-Webster gives the following example of a couch potato: *one who refuses to budge no matter what is needed to be done.*
Synonyms for couch potato: *lazybones, deadbeat, do-nothing, drone, idler, layabout, loafer, lotus-eater, slouch, slug, slugabed, sluggard*

How did this happen?

The United States Department of Agriculture (USDA) is the governing body of our nation that oversees, directs and administers the majority of our food and farm policies. The USDA was established in the 1800s under President Abraham Lincoln's office.

Major changes occurred in the American diet during the Great Depression. Due to the plumping prices of food and the lack of income for families to purchase food, President Roosevelt's administration instituted formal food policy or "Farm Bill"-originally called the *Agriculture Adjustment Act*. This was the first official piece of legislation that provided price controls to encourage farmers to keep producing or growing food and helped to maintain a cost of living for farmers and also help control food prices for the consumers.

The Farm Bill has evolved into a major piece of legislation that is critical to the health and well being of all Americans as well as the ecological integrity of our country (and planet!). Today's Farm bill *sets the rules of the game, influencing not only what we eat, but also who grows it, under what conditions and how much it costs.*[19] It includes legislation that influences public health and nutrition, through the national school lunch program and Supplemental Nutrition Assistance Program or SNAP (food stamps); Wall Street and domestic finances, through the buying and selling of commodity crops that are manufactured and owned by corporations; and energy and climate change, through the way we harvest foods and maintain livestock using fossil fuel, pesticides and how we manage our waste.

The USDA and Farm Bills also provide legislation that defines the scope and duties of Land Grant colleges and universities. These institutions were- and are today! - a major player in food and farming Research & Development (R&D). It is through the USDA that R&D created:

- Synthetic fertilizer
- Genetically Modified Organisms or GMOs
- Frozen foods
- Soy products
- The many, many uses of CORN!

Certain commodity crops developed into major surpluses (that means money) for the United States and other international governments and businesses. Corn and soybeans being two major sources of agriculture income. Since commodities crops bring in the most money, farmers were and are today encourages to produce only those products. This is part of the domino effect on the condition of our environmental crisis: soil erosion, deforestation, water and air pollution, etc.

All other "food" -fruits and vegetables- is considered "specialty crops." AND the majority of these specialty crops do not receive any federal subsidies or support for growing and harvesting.

Fruits and veggies are expensive to grow. There is an increased labor costs: people are needed to care and pick or harvest these foods as they are easily damaged and do not have long shelf lives. Specialty food crops need to be rotated to support good use of soil and to replenish minerals in the soil, so more land is needed to grow these crops.

More and more farmers are discouraged from growing specialty crops if they want to earn a living. Especially since commodity crops like corn, soy and wheat are heavily subsidized, giving farmers a steady income even if they are unable to grow these crops due to weather or a glut of commodities in the market.

Commodity crops like corn have many uses beyond our summer corn-on-the-cob or morning bowl of Cornflakes. Manufacturers are able to "create" both fuel (ethanol) and food (i.e. high fructose corn syrup) from corn. Subsequently, Synthetically made foods and food additives like high fructose corn syrup have become the mainstay of the American diet.

The importance of eating a balanced diet has been a focus of our governance structure for the past 100 years. Food guides provide a conceptual framework for why we eat and what we should eat in order to get the nutrients needed to sustain our lives.

One of the first tasks of the USDA was to develop a scientific-based guideline of good eating for the American public. One of the first formal conversations about the American diet was published in 1894: *The Tables of Food Importance and Dietary Standards for the U.S. Population.* [20] These tables provided the recommendations for the average amount of total calories needed for the average American male, and included specific calorie counts for proteins and unspecified amounts for fats, carbohydrates, vitamins and minerals.[21]

In 1914, the first formal "food guide" was published. Food was categorized into five groups based on the type of foods and the nutrition they provided: milk and milk products; cereals; vegetables and fruits; fats and fat foods; and sugar and sugary foods.

In 1921-23, the USDA's *How to select foods guide*, enhanced the 1914 food guide publication by providing additional recommendations for families to select foods that were high in nutrient value.

The economic challenges of the Great Depression of the 1930s influenced the food guide recommendations in order to support families who had less income to purchase good quality foods. The food guides published during this era, emphasized shopping tips and the "amount of food to buy and use in a week at four cost levels to meet the nutrition needs of people at different ages and income levels.[22] The food guides during this period also emphasized the importance of eating "protective" foods- those high in certain nutrients like calcium, and vitamin A & C. The concept for supporting families' dietary choices through economic hardship continues today. The USDA's Thrifty Food Plan, for example, was developed to provide SNAP (food stamp) recipients with shopping tips to support nutritious eating on a low income.[23]

In 1941, the first "official" guidelines known as the Food and Nutrition Board of the National Academy of Science published the "recommended daily allowances" for foods. Foods continued to be divided into groupings and specific recommendations were provided about the daily intake of nine essential nutrients and what foods provided them. The nine essential nutrients included were: protein; the fat-soluble vitamins and minerals (iron, calcium, vitamin A & D); "B" vitamins (thiamin, riboflavin and niacin); and ascorbic acid (Vitamin C).

Throughout the balance of the 20th century, the USDA continue to update and revised their food guidance along with the new evidence provided by research, scientific studies, the changing American population health demographics, the state of the economy and the focus of the federal food and farm policy.

The domino effect of increasing commodity crop production on the development of fast food ingredients and the overall morbidity of the population's health- especially in weight gain, obesity and food related diseases- urged the USDA, the Department of Health and Human Services as well as the National Institutes on Health to focus national food guidance on not only recommending the types of food to eat in order to assure proper essential nutrient intake, yet also to include recommendations on foods not to eat or to be eaten in moderation. [24]

S.A.D.- Standard American Diet

Even though the USDA recommends that we need to eat five servings of vegetables and fruits everyday, there is no legislation or policy that support the production of these foods. Current food policy supports foods that are cheap and plentiful- fast foods- lacking the essential nutrients we need to maintain good health. *According to a 2006 USDA study, if Americans increased their consumption of fruits and vegetables to meet the USDA dietary recommendations, the U.S. would need an additional 13 million acres of 'specialty crops.'* [25]

There has been a lot of medical research that supports a direct link between eating processed foods and many modern diseases like cancer, hypertension and obesity.

Couch Potato Syndrome & the S.A.D. Diet

Standard American Diet

S = Sodium and Sugar

A = Additives

D = diet-related diseases

- Diabetes
- Gout
- Hypertension/CVD
- Arthritis/ Autoimmune
- Cancers

Recently, scientists found another disturbing link between eating processed foods and developing dementia and Alzheimer's.[26] This new research establishes the relationship of insulin resistance and diabetes to the degeneration of brain cells. Brain cell death is the process for developing dementia and Alzheimer's. These current studies also indicate that younger Americans are beginning to suffer for early signs of dementia and may ultimately develop Alzheimer's. The more junk food we eat over time, the greater our exposure to preservatives and additives like sodium nitrate that affects insulin production and absorption causing a diabetic state in the brain that ultimately leads to Alzheimer's. [27]

Now that we have explored a brief history of some of the environmental impacts on our current health and lifestyle, let us take a deeper look into the body-mind connection.

REFLECTION QUESTION

Take a moment to recall the foods that you ate over the last 24 hours. Write them down. Does your diet reflect the USDA RDA or the S.A.D. diet?

III.

THE MIND-BODY CONNECTION REVISITED- YOUR TWO BRAINS

We consider the mind to be housed in the brain, just like we consider love to be housed in the heart.

Both the mind and love are energetic aspects of your life. Yet they are connected to your physical body as well.

The mind is considered to be a source of emotions. The central nervous system (CNS) is the organ system responsible for the brain and the transmission of information throughout the body. One thought will trigger many physiological responses in your body thanks to the CNS including the sensations of pleasure and pain that keeps you alive and well.

The Gastro-intestinal or digestive system also has a system of neurons – a "brain" -of it's own.

The Enteric Nervous System (ENS) has over 100 million neurotransmitters that are spread throughout the length of your digestive tract, approximately the same number of neurotransmitter cells found in your brain. Actually, the total amount of nerve cells in your gut is greater than the total number of nerves connecting the rest of your body to your brain, therefore the "gut" brain can act independent of the brain in your skull.

The amazing human body developed these two brains during conception. The Vagus Nerve- longest nerve cell in your body- connects both the CNS and the ENS together and this connection allows for communication between your two brains.

Consider the human body in the likeness of a tree. The roots of the tree are like the enteric nervous system: many strands converging to give nourishment to the whole tree or body.

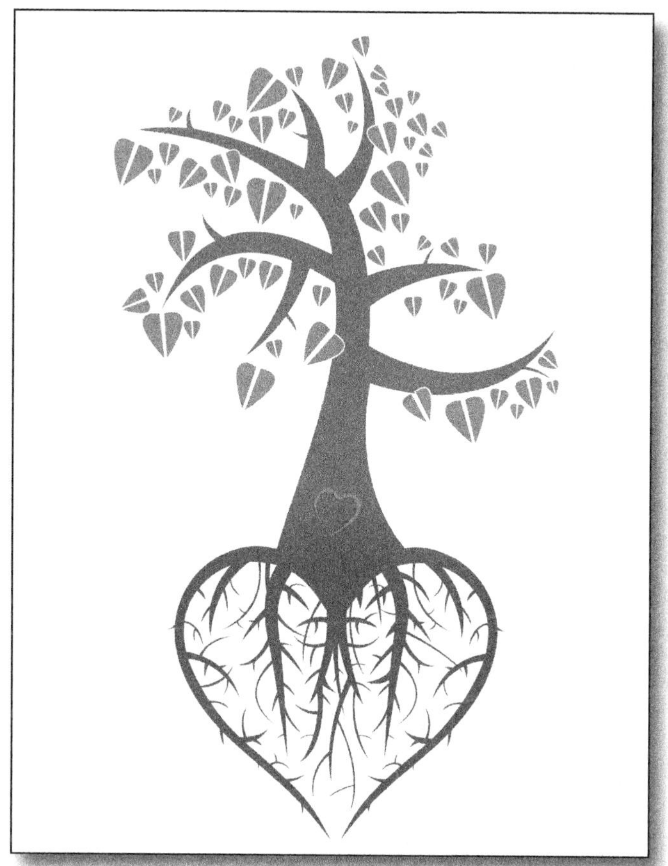

The Branches of the tree is like our brain or central nervous system- always thinking or diverging away from the core to explore life and learn more.
The two are connected to and by the trunk of the body- thus the mind-body connection!

Having a "gut" reaction to a thought or encounter, or getting irritated after eating certain foods explains how your two brains interact with one another and how they may influence your emotions.

How does this relate to our modern lifestyle choices?

The Stress Response

If you recall, STRESS is one of the factors that influence the WELLNESS CONTINUUM.

STRESS is an activity that affects both "brains": CNS and ENS. Here's how:

Stress response in the Central Nervous System

Hormones are chemical substances produced in your body that have a specific effect on the activity of a certain organ or organ systems.

Major hormones- like cortisol, insulin and thyroid stimulating hormone- are key to maintaining stability and regulation of body systems. We cannot live without them. Other hormones- like estrogens, progesterone and testosterone- also support the regulation of specific body systems; however fluctuate in importance over your lifetime.

A primary hormone system in your body is called the Hypothalamus Pituitary Adrenal Axis or "HPA Axis." The HPA Axis helps regulate functions such as your body temperature, digestion, immune system, mood, sexuality and energy usage. It is also a major part of the system that controls your reaction to stress, trauma and injury.

The Emotional Response

Emotions are directly related to the same endocrine or hormone system that influences your stress response and are therefore influenced by both brains. Have you noticed that eating certain foods can effect how you feel? Eating foods that contain caffeine can make you feel energetic or even irritated. Eating sugary foods can make you feel happy and then suddenly drowsy or sleepy after an hour or so.

Why We Crave

We may associate an emotional response to certain foods as cravings. Craving is a strong desire to consume a food or substance.[28] This desire is your physical response to dealing with many of the emotions or feelings you have throughout the day and course of your life.

Below are a few examples of why we crave certain foods:

- De-stress = pain relief (emotional or physical)
- Security= nourishment, love
- Satisfaction= achievement, fulfillment
- Sensuality = pleasure, comfort
- Systematic= desire created through advertisements/ market driven

If your two brains are linked together physiologically, then it makes sense that they would also be linked energetically.
How many folks do you know stop eating when they are upset?
How many folks do you know eat more when they get upset?
How many folks do you know eat when they are happy? Angry, Frustrated?

Interesting too, your "brains" build memories. So an emotion that was "satisfied" by a particular food you ate while you are experiencing that emotion, becomes a memory that relates food to a feeling. If you experience that particular emotion over and over again and you feel the need to comfort yourself, almost unconsciously you may reach for a particular food that made the feeling or emotion go away.

Lastly, we must consider that our cravings are greatly influenced by ADVERTISING. Fast food ads are everywhere! Television, radio, websites such as Facebook, MSN, Yahoo and LinkIn, neighborhood build boards, airports, train stations, buses, subways...everywhere! Virtually impossible to avoid, the impact is understandable: an increase desire to eat at fast food restaurants and the increase in sales for fast food corporations.

REFLECTION QUESTION

Describe one way you cope with stress. How does your coping strategy influence your eating?

IV.

TOOLS TO INCREASE OUR AWARENESS FOR EATING HEALTHIER

With this basic understanding of: how the food system work; and the body-mind connection to why we eat the way we do, what can we do to make the changes necessary for a healthier lifestyle?

First, let's consider the guidelines that are available to assist us.

- The USDA Food Pyramid and My Plate
- Finding hidden calories that are causing excessive weight gain
- Reading food labels
- Organic versus conventional eating
- The Diet Plan Market

From Pyramid to Plate

> *The evils of overeating may not be felt at once, but sooner or later they are sure to appear—perhaps in an excessive amount of fatty tissue, perhaps in general debility, perhaps in actual disease.*
>
> -Wilbur Olin Atwater, USDA 1902[29]

The Food Pyramid- an adaption of a visual dietary guideline concept initially developed in Sweden- was revised over a 13-year period (1992 -2005) to further provide guidance on the types of foods within each of the five major food group categories. It also provides recommendations for the amount of foods to eat daily in each of these food groups and highlights practical guidance for developing good lifestyle habits:

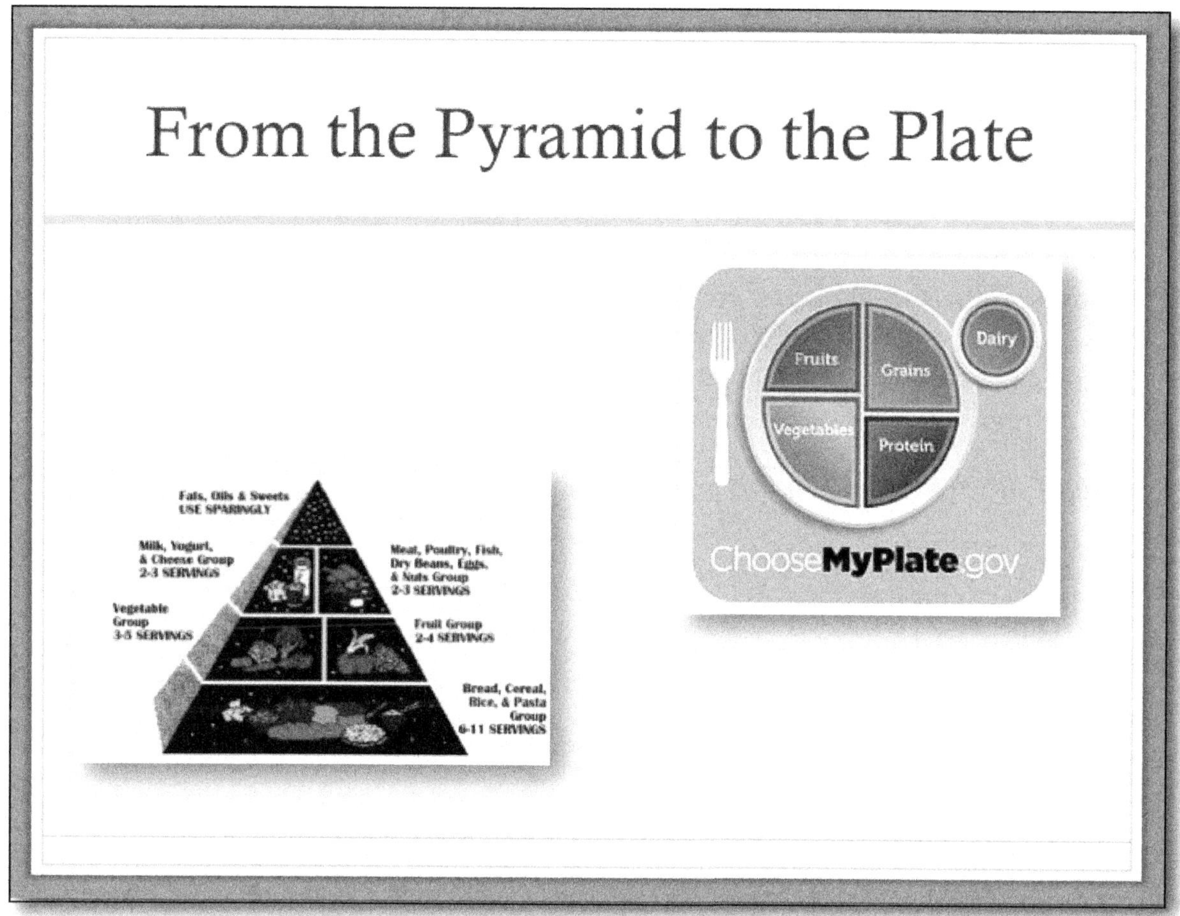

- Eat a variety of foods
- Maintain a healthy weight
- Eat a low fat, low cholesterol diet
- Eat lots of fruits, vegetables and grains
- Eat sugar, salt, sodium in moderation
- Consume alcoholic beverages in moderation

Why the plate?

In 2010, the USDA published the *Healthy Eating Guidelines 2010*. Because of the epidemic proportion of diet-related illnesses facing America, a new concept to support healthy eating was developed: *My Plate*. The idea behind *My Plate* is to provide a visual framework for eating foods by groups and in proper portions. Four basic food groups are "visual" on the plate and by portion size: 1/2 of the plate's portion is for vegetables and fruits; ¼ of the plate is for protein (meat, poultry, fish, legumes, nuts); ¼ of the plate is from whole grain products. The fourth food grouping is visualized as by a "glass" sits aside *My Plate* to represent dairy intake. Helping Americans "see" what their food plate should look like for each meal may assure that they are getting the recommended daily nutrient requirements and decrease the amount of empty calories and fatty foods since these are not visible on the plate.

There are many variations of the "pyramid" and "plate" designed by folks who are trying to emphasize their ideal dietary strategies (i.e. macrobiotics, veganism, vegetarianism). These visuals aides may be useful if you are considering adopting one of these diet strategies. You can find them by researching the web.

Hidden Calories: It's all in the portion size

The portion sizes of foods we eat today have really been "supersized." This is the main culprit in our weight gain.

The example shown below is based on the increase in the size of these average foods and the increase in the amount of calories and fats in the same foods we eat today.

The *Old* column stands for portion sizes of 20 + years ago. The *New* column is the average calorie per gram in today's version of the food.

<u>Muffins</u>- The increase in the size of an average muffin at *Dunkin Donuts* has doubled over the past two decades. The average muffin at *Dunkin Donuts* has about 200 more calories than their most sugary donut.

<u>Bagels</u>- An "old" style bagel represents something like the old Lender's bagels (they were a wee bit bigger than the mini bagels we eat today) as compared to a bagel purchased at *Dunkin Donuts* or *Starbucks* of today. The calories noted in the "new" column do not include adding cream cheese!

<u>Coffee</u>- back in the day, a "regular" coffee was 8 ounces of black coffee with a little milk and sugar. Today, the average regular cup of Joe consumed may be a Grande-Mocha-whatnot with whipped cream or other sweeteners.

<u>House salad</u>- Twenty years ago, the average restaurant served a "house salad" that included romaine or iceberg lettuce, a tomato, cucumber and some olive oil. Today, fast food restaurants like McDonald's are attempting to jump on the healthy food lifestyle but haven't quite got it correct. The standard salad at Micky D's: mixed greens, croutons,

Hidden Calories?

It's all in the portion size

	Old	New
Muffins	200 cal/7g	590 cal/24g
Bagels	200 cal	400 cal
Coffee	120 cal/2g	490 cal/26g
"house" Salad	153 cal/2g	660 cal/51g
Wine	100 cal	300 cal

bacon bits, grilled chicken and high calorie dressing. This salad served with *Newman's Own* dressing has more calories than the *Big Mac*!

Wine- In the old days, the average person may have consumed one, 4 ounce glass of wine, sipped after dinner. Today, the average person consumes ½ a bottle alone at one sitting.

An easy way to eat fewer calories is to cut down the portion size.

Reading Food Labels

A good way to understand portion sizes is by reading the nutritional food label on the products that you buy. All food labels provide some basic information about the food product: serving size; number of calories; percentage of macronutrients (fats, carbohydrates and proteins); percentage of micronutrients (vitamins and minerals); and the

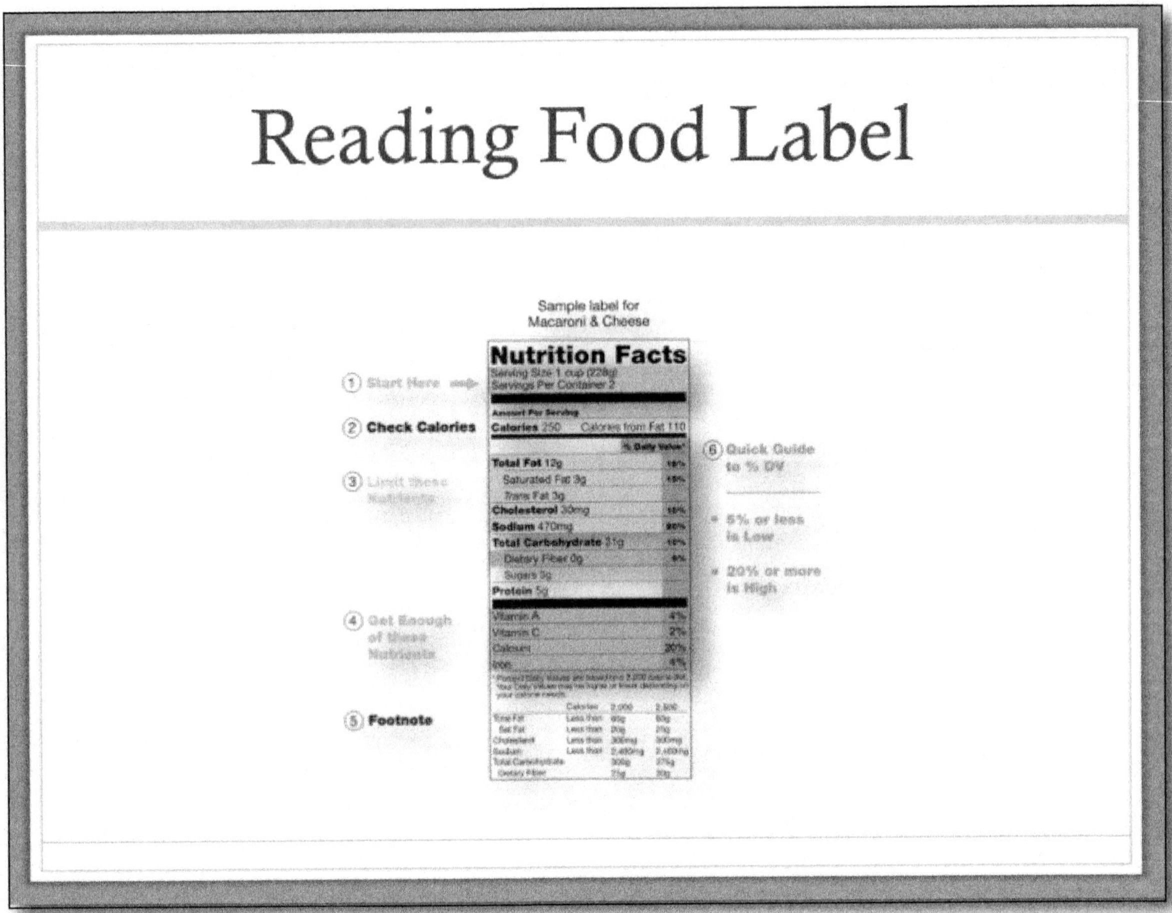

USDA's recommended daily allowance ("daily value") for those macro and micro nutrients listed in the product's ingredients. The food and Drug Administration's (FDA) rule of thumb for considering a food as "low fat" or "high fat" is based on the percentage of fat per the recommended Daily Value (DV). If the fat content of a food is 5% or less of the DV, the food is considered low fat. If the fat content of a food is 20% or more of the DV, the food is considered high fat.[30]

The serving size is listed on the top of the food label (see example). The serving size is very important because it tells you the portion size that the other information provided on the food label relates to. For example, the food label above is for a box of instant macaroni and cheese. The "servings per container" is for two cups. The serving size is for one cup not two. Therefore, if you eat the entire box of Mac and cheese then you are getting double the amount of calories, fats, protein, sodium, etc. listed on the food label.

Reading Food labels

Although the Food and Drug Administration (FDA) monitors "Good Manufacturing Practices" (GMP) there are loopholes in the regulations that if left uncheck, may lead you to take in more calories and other ingredients than you anticipated.

For example, certain ingredients like Trans fat that weighs 0.5 grams or less, may not be included on the food label. So if your favorite snack advertises, "zero fat" or "fat free" on the label, read the list of ingredients carefully.

The language used in the list of ingredients may also seem vague or a little deceiving. By definition, the FDA defines a food or ingredient as "natural" when an ingredient or food is "derived from a natural source."[31] However, some natural-styled synthetic ingredients can also be labeled as "natural". For example, ascorbic acid, which is vitamin C, is derived naturally from oranges, is also made synthetically in a lab.

Lastly, food manufacturers changed their ingredients and product formulas more often than we might think. So read the Nutrition Fact Panel each time you buy, especially those products that you like and buy a lot.

The following is an example of commonly used ingredients in processed foods. The FDA maintains a current list of over 3000 ingredients on its database: Everything Added to Food in the United States (EAFUS): *http://www.accessdata.fda.gov/scripts/fcn/fcnNavigation.cfm?rpt=eafusListing*

SUGAR- sucrose, glucose, fructose, sorbitol, mannitol, corn syrup, high fructose corn syrup, Saccharin, aspartame, sucralose, acesulfame potassium, neotame

FAT- olestra, cellulose gel, carrageenan, poly dextrose, modified food starch, microparticulated egg white protein, guar gum, xanthan gum, whey protein concentrate

PRESERVATIVES- ascorbic acid, citric acid, sodium benzonte, calcium sorbate, potassium sorbate, BHA, BHT, EDTA, tocopherol (vitamin E)

ADDITIVES- in 1958, Congress amended the Federal Food, Drug and Cosmetic Act. The 1958 Food Additive Amendment defines and regulates "any substance intentionally added to food is a food additive and subject to pre-market approval by the FDA unless the use of the substance is Generally Recognized As Safe (GRAS).[32]

The FDA categorizes food additives into two groups:

Group 1: Prior-sanctioned substances. Additives the FDA and USDA deemed "safe" prior to the 1958 amendment. These include sodium nitrate and potassium nitrate.

Group 2: GRAS or Generally Recognized As Safe ingredients by the FDA and USDA based on their historical use prior to the 1958 amendment or current scientific evidence. Examples include: salt, sugar, spices, vitamins, monosodium glutamate (MSG)

Additional resources for understanding food labels and ingredients are included in the RESOURCE section on the guide.

Is Organic Better?

Eating the highest quality foods that are free of toxins and chemicals that may ill effect your health overtime is best. Finding sources of high quality foods can be a challenge for many reasons: availability and costs probably being two of the most challenging reasons.

Organic foods are whole foods and animal products that are grown, harvested and preserved without the use of chemicals. The earth that organic foods are grown in does not contain any chemical fertilizer or non-organic matter. Organic foods are not sprayed with pesticides or other chemicals nor are manipulated in any way by chemicals or non-organic matter in order to increase their shelf life: including the transit time from farm to store.

Conventional foods are foods and animal products that are grown in farming areas or gardens that do use chemical fertilizers, pesticides and additives to increase their shelf life.

The chart below provides a comparison of organic or non-organic (conventional) foods.

Truth in labeling. For foods to be truly organic, they must be grown, harvested and preserved without chemicals. Trickier still, is for animal products to be truly considered organic, because the manner in which they are raised- where animals are housed, what they eat and how they get to eat it- also weighs into the organic label equation. Producing organic foods and raising organic-based animal products is expensive, time consuming and requires a lot of land. Without the use of pesticides, chemical fertilizers, preservatives and -in the case of animals- hormones or other growth enhancing medicines, organics

Is Organic Better?

CONVENTIONAL	ORGANIC
Apply chemical fertilizer to promote plant growth.	Apply natural fertilizers, such as manure or compost, to feed soil and plants.
Spray synthetic insecticides to reduce pests and disease.	Spray pesticides from natural sources; use beneficial insects and birds, mating disruption or traps to reduce pests and disease.
Use synthetic herbicides to manage weeds.	Use environmentally-generated plant-killing compounds; rotate crops, till hand weed or mulch to manage weeds.
Give animals antibiotics, growth hormones and medications to prevent disease and spur growth.	Give animals organic feed and allow them access to the outdoors. Use preventive measures-such as rotational grazing, a balanced diet and clean housing-to help minimize disease.

Chart source[33]

have a short shelf- life. We consumers as well as the grocers who sell us these products must use/sell them quickly or risk the loss of product and money.

The current debate with organic labeling includes producers who may use some of the organic standards like not using pesticides but not following some of the other standards like using chemical fertilizers in the soil that they grow in. These producers still consider their foods and animal products to be organic, even though all of the organic standards are not met. In these instances, food packaging may read, “Includes organic ingredients” or “naturally grown” however reading all of the ingredients will prove the efficacy of the organic standards.

V.

WHAT'S THE BEST DIET PLANS ON THE MARKET TODAY?

Weight-loss is a $240 billion business[34]. With so much money to be made how can we best choose the best diet on the market? Is it *Weight Watchers*, *Jenny Craig*, *Atkins*, Vegan, *American Diabetes Associations'*, *or* Vegetarianism?

To consider which is the best diet for you depends on some key factors.

Keys to a Good Diet
Balance of Macro-Nutrients
Supports Optimal GI Function
Encourages Exercise
Group Support

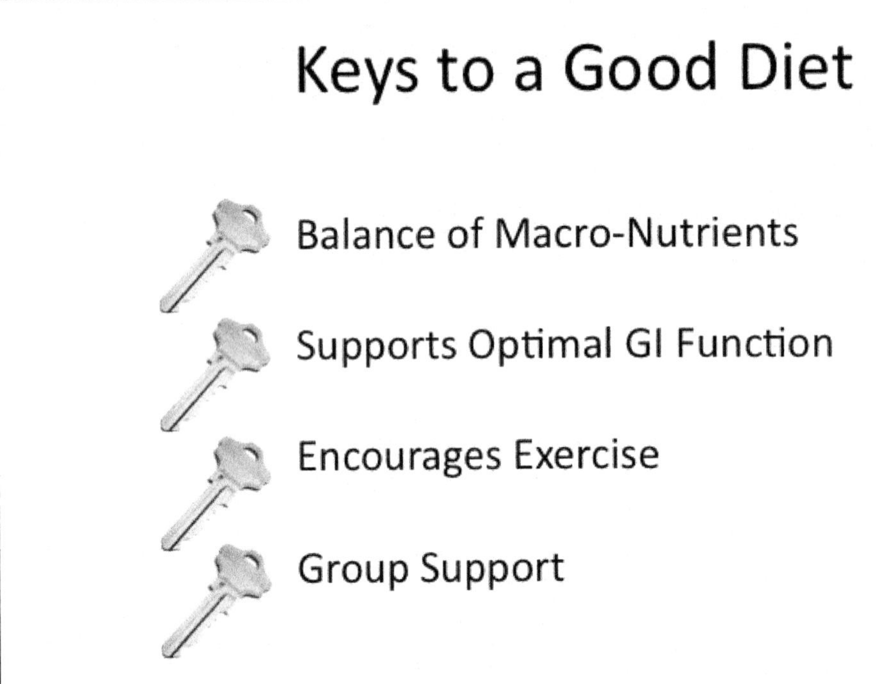

The majority of packaged "diet" strategies are basically the same with a variation on: the types of suggested foods to eat that is usually based on the writer's opinion; personal experience; and (hopefully) their subjective interpretation of scientific research.

If you decide to follow a commercial diet, consider the following key elements in the package that you purchase (NOTE: the following suggestions are the minimum standards of a quality diet plan!):

Balance of Macro-Nutrients. A good diet, regardless if it's conventional, vegetarian, emphasizes more protein, eating for your blood type, etc., offer balanced menu choices that include high quality sources of foods that contain: essential vitamins and minerals (micronutrients); proteins from both vegetable and animal sources; complex carbohydrates and essential fats from fish and vegetable-based sources.

Supports Optimal GI function. Healthy weight loss begins with proper digestion. What you eat, how you metabolize certain foods, how nutrients are stored or assimilated in your body to support your health all depends on optimal gastro-intestinal (GI) function. When considering one of the commercial diets, be sure to look for how their diet addresses maintaining good digestion including daily elimination of foods.

Encourages Exercise. No diet will be 100% successful without exercise. Your body must expel or use the energy that you fill it up with, otherwise this excess of energy will be stored as fat and you will gain weight. A good commercial diet will encourage you to balance your calorie intake with the amount of energy you use everyday.

Group Support. Striving to change your lifestyle is easier with a supportive community around you. The success of *Weight Watchers* over the past 40 years has been strongly influenced by the group and peer support built into the diet and lifestyle strategies. You don't have to do it alone. Having champions in your corner encouraging you will keep you motivated.

Are diet foods good for you?

Many diet plans offer pre-packaged meals to support their weight loss maintenance programs. But diet plans like *Healthy Choice, Smart Ones* and *Eating Right* meals are expensive, with the average cost of $5 per entrée. *Budget Gourmet* is less expensive, with an average entrée cost of $2 but the portion sizes are smaller. These pre-packaged meals also contain lots of artificial flavors, sugar and sodium and not enough daily fiber that may be adding more health risk than the diet may be worth. Because these plans are designed to help you loose weight, the portion sizes, like in *Lean Cuisine*, are low in calories. Drastically reducing your daily intake of calories can leave you feeling hungrier and cause you to snack more. Ultimately you end up eating more calories than you realize!

You can make your own diet plan by selecting better choices for your meals and by eating less of what you choose.

For example, if you choose to eat a pre-package diet meal, have it for lunch or dinner, but not both. Be sure to eat a high protein breakfast like a hard-boiled egg and a slice of whole grain toast with peanut butter and a piece of fruit. Bring healthy snacks with you to work or school like fruit, vegetable slices (carrots, fresh green beans, and green leafy salad) or nuts. Drink lots of water throughout the day and be sure to find 30 minutes for exercise.

Five Great Reasons to Drink Water

Water may not seem as exciting a beverage as soda or juice, but it is a key ingredient for your diet that should be consumed everyday.

Here are five great reasons to drink water everyday:[35]

1. Water keeps us alive. You can live for about a month without food, but only about a week without water.
2. Water helps you maintain healthy body weight by increasing metabolism and regulating your appetite.
3. Water helps increase your energy. The most common cause of daytime fatigue is actually mild dehydration.
4. Water improves your health by flushing out wastes and bacteria that can cause disease.
5. Water is the main way that vitamins and nutrients get circulated around your body.

Barriers to Living a Healthier Lifestyle

Based on the information just shared, it is easy to understand how we can become overwhelmed by the choices we make everyday to live a long healthy life. There are many forces influencing our choices and many choices to make. Changing our lifestyle is a challenge. The ways in which we live have developed into habits and habits are hard to break. The way we think- as we previously discussed- influences how we act. This too adds to developing behavior patterns or habits.

Sometimes, we find "legitimate" excuses for not sticking to our change plans: not enough time, not enough money or other pressing obligations. If you can stand back from these

Barriers to Healthy Living Choices: Imagined/Real

IMAGINED	REAL
Time	Fear
Money	Discipline
Obligations	Motivation

excuses emotionally, more than likely you find that your reasons are more imagined than realistic. The strength of the human mind is such that it can create whatever reality it wishes to imagine. With this ability, you also "will" or focus your mind on activities and things that you want and with this very intention are successful at achieving the things you focused your intention to do.

For example, you may feel that you live on a limited budget and cannot afford the cost of foods that would better nourish and sustain your health. But, if you have a craving for something that you really enjoy, like eating out at the Cheesecake Factory once a week, you "find" the funds to do this because you like it, the experience satisfies you and therefore you focus your intention on assuring that the money is available to participate.

Overcoming the barriers to living a healthier lifestyle begins with being realistic about the challenges that are stopping you. Your fears, lack of discipline and lack of motivation are real obstacles that affect your mind and emotions and subsequently your physical ability to move out and actively make the change.

REFLECTION QUESTIONS

1. Review the list of active feelings in the *Emotional Hierarchy Chart.* As you read each one, close your eyes and imagine the feeling that you associate with each word. You may begin to notice that the words listed above the neutral line tend to make you feel more relaxed. Notice how the words below the neutral line make you feel. Are

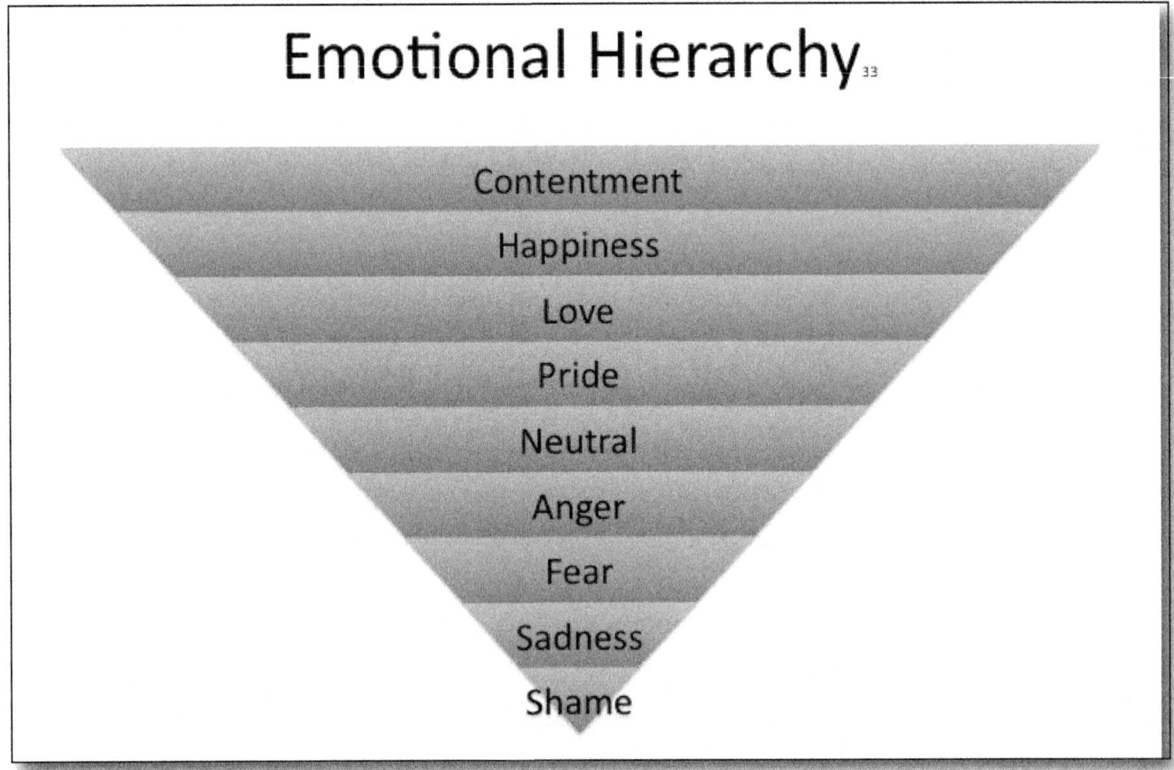

these feelings the same as the ones you experience reading the words above the neutral line?

Imagine now, the types of decisions you would make experiencing the feelings that these words are associated with in your heart and mind. How successful would you be trying a new lifestyle change activity while feeling content or happy? How successful would you be while feeling angry, fearful or ashamed?

Being able to identify how you associate certain words with your feelings is the beginning of a self-study practice that will increase your awareness about yourself. Successful lifestyle changes come along with an increased awareness of self.

2. Before choosing what to eat, take an emotional check-in. If your feeling experience is above the neutral line, then you are probably making a better choice about what to eat. If your feeling experience is below the neutral line, then wait before make a food choice and take a few moments to uncover why you are feeling what you are feelings. What have you been doing up to the point of reaching for food? What thoughts may have triggered the emotion? How would eating your foods of choice satisfy the feelings you are experiencing?

VI.

SIMPLE STEPS FOR A HEALTHIER LIFESTYLE

Simple Steps For a Healthier Lifestyle
1. Follow My Plate
2. Skip Snacks
3. Drink More Water
4. Exercise- the best excuse for eating more is because you are using more fuel!

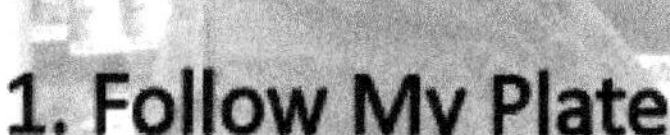

Four basic principles for weight loss are to:

1. Follow the *My Plate* pattern and be sure that the plate you fill at every meal has the basic foods and portion sizes as illustrated on *My Plate* graphic (See resources)

2. Skip snacks. Snacks add additional calories to your daily calorie intake. When you snack, you tend not to pay attention to portion sizes either.

3. Drink more water. Earlier on in this workbook, is a list of 5 good reasons to drink water (see page 30). Approximately 60% of your body is composed of water.

Most of us don't drink enough water and are dehydrated. Your body needs to replenished water everyday.

4. Exercise! The best excuse for eating more calories is because your body needs to use more fuel. Exercise requires fuel. Sitting requires very little fuel. Later on in the workbook, there is an entire section devoted to exercise so read on! (See section VIII)

Strategies for developing a healthy lifestyle routine

The four basic principles for weight loss will put you on the right track, however additional strategies are needed to really be successful at losing weight and moving towards a healthier lifestyle.

> *Being healthy means all things working in accordance with its nature, aim and purpose.*

Strategies for Developing a Healthy Lifestyle Routine
Self-Study
Discipline
YOU!
Overcome Habits
Change Eating Patterns

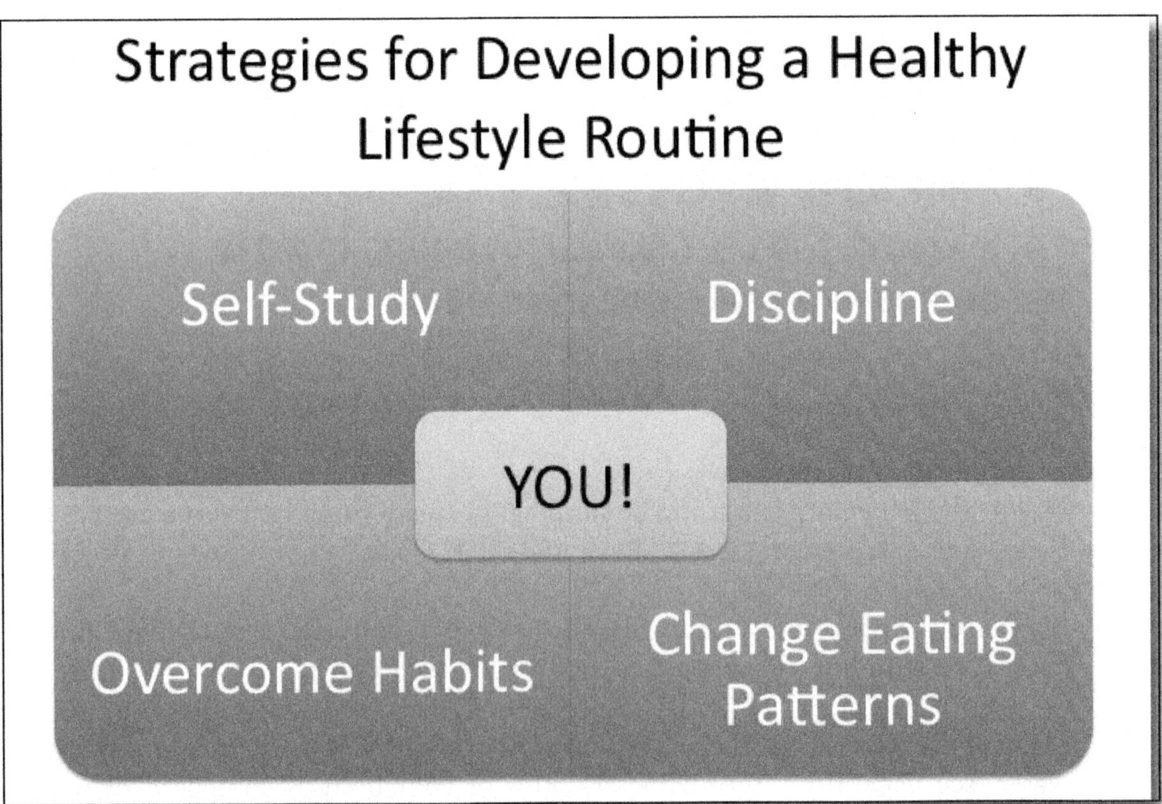

Self-study. Did you know that you are an interesting and fascinating person? Check yourself out! You will learn a lot about humanity by turning your lens inward. There are many ways to do this. For many people, self-study is supported by a spiritual or religious practice. For others, it may be listening to or reading books by motivational self-help practitioners. Movement practices like yoga, Qi Gong, Tai Chi, martial arts, dance, etc., can also be a process of self-study as you learn how your body responses to certain movements.

Regardless of what type of self-study choice you choose, it is essential to building your will. A strong will is essential to becoming more disciplined. It is difficult to take on a discipline for any real length of time without understanding how and why it affects the self. Taking on any discipline through action only, is usually short lived because if you do not truly understand you current emotions, thoughts, patterns and behaviors and what inside and outside forces influence them, you will return to your old ways because your old ways are comfortable. You taking the step to participate in the *Healthy Weight, Healthy You!* workshop series is a step towards self-study. Keep going.

Establish a routine. Routines help us to function daily. They represent patterns of behavior and activities that support our lifestyles. From the time we are born, routines are established. Newborns will habituate to feeding and sleeping times and subsequently influence the routines of their parents. As we grow through life, our systems of education and work continue to guide us with routines that organize our day.

Routines are really forms of discipline. They are plans in action. As you begin to set new lifestyle goals, consider the action steps you need to do everyday to reach your goals. If you can find one or two activities to do DAILY that will support your goal, you will be successful. Establish a routine (discipline) to become AWARE of HOW you are feeling BEFORE you choose to eat! One excellent activity to practice daily is using the *Emotional Hierarchy Chart* (see page 32) before choosing your meals or deciding to snack. Not only will this activity support your healthy weight goals, it will also help you cultivate a desire to overcome emotional responses that keep you in your not-so-good habits.

Change your eating patterns. Before beginning another diet, do an assessment of your current eating patterns. For one week, write down meals: everything you eat, the time of day that you ate it and how you felt before, during and after you ate. Notice the patterns in your current diet. Write down the changes you would like to see in your current eating pattern. Set a goal to implement one change per month. Start slow. For example, the first monthly goal may be to eat smaller portion sizes of carbs that you like (pasta, rice, potatoes, breads, cakes, cookies, chips). The second monthly goal may be to change your carb food of choice for another type of food, for example, choosing a whole grain like quinoa instead of pasta or rice. Whatever choice you decide to begin with, choose a strategy that will assure your success.

VII.

KITCHEN SCIENCE WISDOM

Our eating habits shape us in ways few of us suspect. The food we eat is vital to both our physical and our mental health. Complementary medicine is rediscovering the close connection between body and mind, and is beginning to look at diet as a critical factor in health maintenance and restoration.36

There was a time in our history that the production and preparation of food was considered a "science" for maintaining good health. Women (mostly) as the central caregiver and nurturer of the home were charged with assuring the health and well-being of her family. Sayings like "old wives tales", or "motherwit" speak to an inner wisdom that women shared and passed down to her family- usually daughters- filled with intuitive practices that supported everyone's well-being. Her kitchen, being the central location in the home, is where this wisdom was practiced.

What is Kitchen Science Wisdom?

The word *Kitchen* comes from an old Latin root that means "to decoct"; or "to extract the flavor or active principle of." The word *Science* comes from the Latin root word meaning "to know." It is "knowledge gained through experience."
Wisdom, then, is the practical application of science. Once we have knowledge of a thing then we are able to put that knowledge into practice through "common sense" and "good judgment."[37]

Kitchen Science Wisdom is the practice of cooking and eating for health and well-being. It is cooking delicious and nutritious meals with the knowledge of balancing nutrients by combining a variety of foods like vegetables, complex carbohydrates and proteins, and using herbs, spices and essential fats (i.e. oils) to enhance the flavor and activate the chemistry or nutrients of the foods to support our health.

How do we put all of this information together in order to help us meet our healthy weight loss goals?

Let's reconsider how we prepare our food.

Back in the day, our grannies knew that certain foods, herbs and spices combined to support our health, well-being and mood.

For example: Chicken Soup. Chicken soup- or any soup really- is one of the best medicinal food recipes that can be found. Why? Because soups combine lots of nutrients in one pot. A typical chicken soups recipe begins with chicken stock- water that has extracted minerals from the boiling chicken. Adding essential vegetables like carrots and tomatoes provides a good source of Vitamin A, C and quercitin: immune boosting nutrients. Potatoes and celery are good sources of fiber, while onions, garlic, basil and thyme provide additional anti-microbial support. Cayenne and salt and indeed flavor enhancers and they also help to disburse all of the other nutrients throughout the entire soup so you get a good dose of vitamins and minerals in every spoon.

Another good example is the beverage of warm milk and cinnamon. Warming milk releases Tryptophan, an enzyme that has a calming effect on the body and enhances sleep. Cinnamon adds a touch of sweetness to the beverage and also helps to balance blood sugar.

Cultural Cooking Styles

There is a lot of research currently being conducted about the impact on the health of populations who move away from their traditional diets and take up the Standard American Diet (S.A.D.). Indigenous communities in India, China, Central & South America and Africa, for example, that traditionally did not suffer from diet-related diseases like diabetes, gout, cancers and obesity are showing pandemics of these diseases that are directly related to their change in dietary choices. What does this say about the state of our health since we live and breathe this type of diet most of our lives?

Every community of people are given their own diet and medicinal plants to support their health- from Europe, to the Arctic north, Antarctic south, North & South Americas, Pacific Islands and Australia- people are given foods that will sustain their lives based on their natural surroundings. People have their own medicine. Living in a "melting pot" culture like we do here in the U.S., most of us have moved away from our traditional diets and are suffering from the impact of the "diet of influence" that the Western diet is gaining a notorious reputation for.

The key to moving towards a more balanced diet and lifestyle, is to look back at our old food preparation traditions and embrace those that we intuitively know will lead us towards a more harmonious life. Also, expanding your diet and trying new things may be worthwhile, especially with ingredients (produce or spices for example) from other traditional cultures that you may not be familiar with.

Taste Sensations

Traditional culinary and health practices like TCM of China, Ayurveda of India, African and Native American healing arts all use the concept of taste to help identify foods and identify the medicinal properties of plants or foods for health.
Most of these traditions observe at least five tastes: sweet, salty, sour, spicy and bitter.

The Five Tastes Defined

Sweet. Sweetness is a taste that is easy to love. It is one of the first tastes that we learn as babies: our mother's milk is sweet and also provides us with the essential nutrients we need as newborns. The sweet taste also represents foods that are high in glucose- brain food- that brings nourishment to our mental abilities and quick energy. Examples of sweet tasting herbs: cinnamon, stevia and sugar cane.

Salty. Salt is the opposite of sweet and therefore balances the sweet taste. These are the two most primitive of taste as sweet alerts us to foods that will bring us quick energy and salt alerts us to foods that will balance electrolyte function (cellular energy balance). Salt and sweet are mainstays of the Standard American Diet (S.A.D.) This makes sense, since most Americans live a fast paced, heady lifestyle and therefore choose foods that are high in sugar and salt. In traditional cuisines, salty herbs were added at the end of the cooking process, to enhance the flavor. Sea salt and seaweed are good sources of salty taste as they also contain other minerals besides just sodium, like calcium, magnesium and potassium.

Sour. Sour tasting foods like lemons, plain yogurt, fermented foods like vinegar and other pickled foods like cucumbers, are another taste that is often use in combination with sweet foods to add harmony. Sour foods and herbs tend to stimulate digestion and therefore help to increase the absorption of vitamins and minerals.

Bitter. The bitter taste is the least appealing taste to most westerners, however usually makes for good medicine. There is nothing like swallowing a "bitter pill" to get healed. Bitter tasting foods like dark green leafy vegetables (spinach, kale, collards and cabbage), black tea, coffee, turmeric and dandelion roots are great examples of foods and spices that support digestive function, act as detoxifiers and natural antibiotics to keep us healthy through the cold seasons.

Spicy. The spicy taste adds the "icing" on top of any great dish. These herbs and spices offer the synergy that completes any menu: dispersing all of the taste that you have been working to blend in your pot so that every spoonful taste delicious.

Spicy foods also support the healing mechanisms of the common cold by clearing sinuses, and promoting sweat and enhancing detoxification. The same "healing" properties that synthetic remedies like Vicks Vapor Rub claim to do.

How to use spices to maximize taste

Nature gives us many herbs that when blended together, brings out the delicious flavors of foods.

Most of the herbs used in western cuisine come in four basic flavors: spicy, sweet, sour and salty. It takes all four flavors mixed together to really enhance foods. So have fun experimenting with taste until you find the perfect blend that fits your taste buds!

TIPS:

1. Be sure to taste each spice first so that you know what it taste like by itself.

2. Start mixing with ¼ teaspoon of each herb. Taste as you go and add a "pinch" of the flavor you want more of. Keep adding a pinch until you've got the perfect flavor for you!

3. Be careful with the Spicy herbs! Start with a pinch. Spicy herbs like cayenne get HOTTER the longer you cook it. A good tip is to add cayenne last- right before the food is done cooking. A pinch of spicy can go a long way.

Here's a sample of different herbs and spices for each of the four flavors:

Four Taste Flavors

SPICY	SWEET	SOUR	SALTY
Cayenne	Cinnamon	Lemon	Garlic
Ginger	Coriander	Onion	Kombu
Basil	Nutmeg	Turmeric	Sea Salt

The following Handouts are available for you in the resource section of the workbook:

- FOOD STAPLES TO KEEP IN YOUR PANTRY
- HOW TO SHOP ON A LOW BUDGET
- A WEEK'S WORTH OF LUNCH MENUS FOR $5/DAY
- SAMPLE RECIPES

VIII.

EXERCISE MOOD & FOOD

Exercise: Early observations

1. Hippocrates (460-370 B.C.)

"If we could give every individual the right amount of nourishment and exercise, not too little and not too much, we would have found the safest way to health"

2. Galen (*A.D. 129-210)*

"Those movements which do not alter respiration are not called exercise"

3. A. Cornelius Celsus (ca.10-60)

"Take exercise: for whilst inaction weakens the body, work strengthens it; the former brings on premature old age, the latter prolongs youth"

4. Hieronymus Mercuralis (1530-1606)

"Exercise is deliberate and planned movement of the human frame, accompanied by breathlessness, and undertaken for the sake of health or fitness..."

Exercise, Defined

What is exercise?
First and foremost, exercise is *DISCIPLINE.* By formal definition, exercise is: *Activity that requires physical or mental exertion, especially when performed to develop or maintain fitness.*"[38]

The meaning of exercise is rooted in the ancient phrase *arek* that means to *hold, contain, or guard*: having high regard for your life means that you exercise in order to take care (hold and guard) what you hold dear!

The evolution of human beings has been a constant quest towards perfection in the use of our body, mind and spirit to sustain life. As we set our minds towards building civilization, our bodies were often used as a "tool" to support the building and maintenance of societies throughout the ages. The 20th century moved most of western civilization into a service-driven industry. We no longer need to use our body as a tool- only our mind! However, the pursuit of intellect has made us sedentary rather than pursuers of higher consciousness that really requires us to use all of our faculties or inherit abilities. The ancient Greeks, Mayans, Native Americans, East Africans and Asians knew the importance of the mind-body-spirit connection and therefore kept physical movement that enhances mind and spirit in the forefront of their traditions. Their success in these realms are why we are re-thinking these traditions and incorporating many of these customs like meditation, yoga and martial arts into our own contemporary lifestyles.

Physiology of Exercise

Any and all physical movement is considered exercise. Certain movements support different aspects of physical, mental and emotional health therefore a variety of movement throughout the day is best practice.

Types of Exercise

Aerobic. Aerobic exercises are fast paced movements that require patterned breathing and increased heart rate. Aerobic exercises support cardiovascular and respiratory functioning and increase mental concentration. Exercising aerobically also improves your mood. Types of aerobic exercise include: jogging/running, walking, swimming, Zumba, Jazzercise, dancing, martial arts, Pilates.

Strength Training. Good bone health and muscle tone begins with strength-based exercises. A lack of strength-based training can lead to hip fractures, osteoporosis, joint pain and weakness. Types of strength-based exercise include: weights, Pilates, Curves, yoga.

Stretching. Lengthening, strengthening and toning muscles, tendons and ligaments require stretch-based movements and exercises. ***Stretching before any other exercise is a good strategy for injury prevention.*** Types of stretch-based exercises include: yoga, Pilates, dancing, martial arts, Qi Gong.

A pitch for yoga!

Being a yoga instructor, I must take a moment to discuss the benefits of this wonderful application.

Yoga is a beautiful getting-to-know yourself practice. Of the multitude of exercise regiments and spiritual protocols known today, yoga provides a personal, practical application for living a holistic lifestyle: uniting the mind, body and spirit.

The term "Yoga" describes a general category of spiritual and philosophical traditions within many Eastern cultures. Here in the United States, the Hatha Yoga tradition is most well-known and studied. Hatha Yoga is a physical movement practice of postures (or *Asanas)* that guides the practitioner into a deeper self awareness, moving the body in relation to the breath.

Hatha Yoga has therapeutic benefits for the body. Of its many gifts, yoga strengthens and tones the muscles, supports healthy digestive function, decreases blood pressure, stimulates circulation, supports the central nervous system and detoxifies the lymphatic system. If you have not exercised in a while, yoga is a good practice to begin with. Look for a Beginner's or Gentle Hatha Yoga class before gradually moving to a more advanced yoga class like Vinyasa (Flow) or Bikram/Hot yoga.

Exercise and mood

Exercise has a direct effect on your emotions and mood. Moving your body stimulates your nervous system and helps to regulate the APA Axis (stress response) that was discussed in section III. Many athletes and folks who exercise regularly speak about hitting a "zone": a point during their practice that endorphins are release that helps them to feel euphoric. Exercising regularly can also support your ability to rest and sleep more soundly.

Exercise and Detoxification

Your body needs to detoxify from pollutants that are present in the environment as well as in the foods we need. Several organs in your body act as blood filters and support the detoxification process. Your lymphatic system also supports detoxification and acts as a drainage system moving wastes away from your blood. Exercising supports this process because it increases blood circulation and helps to expedite the flow of blood through all of your filters: liver, kidneys, lungs and heart. In addition, exercising daily helps to regulate the amount of sugar in your blood.

Exercise and Diet

Exercise helps to control your weight by using extra calories that otherwise would be stored as fat. The number of calories you eat and use each day controls your body weight. Everything you eat contains calories, and everything you do uses calories, including sleeping, breathing, and digesting food. Any physical activity in addition to what you normally do will use extra calories.

Regular exercise is an important part of effective weight loss and weight maintenance. It also can help prevent several diseases and improve your overall health. It does not matter what type of physical activity you perform—sports, planned exercise, household chores, yard work, or work-related tasks—all are beneficial.

Studies show that even the most inactive people can live healthier by doing 30 minutes or more of physical activity per day. Whether you are trying to lose weight or maintain it, you should understand the important role of physical activity and include it in your lifestyle. Exercising everyday supports your discipline! Establishing an exercise routine can support your diet goals too.

Control your weight loss by balancing eating with exercise

Simple truths to consider:

- When you eat more calories than you need to perform your day's activities, your body stores the extra calories and you gain weight.

- When you eat fewer calories than you use, your body uses the stored calories and you lose weight.
- When you eat the same amount of calories as your body uses, your weight stays the same.

Any type of physical activity you choose to do—strenuous activities such as running or aerobic dancing or moderate-intensity activities such as walking or household work—will increase the number of calories your body uses. The key to successful weight control and improved overall health is making physical activity a part of your daily routine.

Calories Burned During Exercise[39]

Calories Burned During Exercise[37]

Exercise/Activity for 1 Hour	Calories Burned!
Housework (cleaning, dusting, vacuuming)	148 kcal
Carrying infants; young children	177 kcal
Playing actively with your children	360 kcal
Low impact aerobics	295 kcal
Moderate walking	220 kcal
Sitting; light office work	89 kcal

Tips for establishing an Exercise Routine

Daily Exercise Routine

Work Day	Weekend
AM: 15 minute workout 12 oz water Protein-rich breakfast	AM: Protein-rich Breakfast 60 minute mixed exercise 12 oz water
Lunchtime: micronutrient-rich lunch 10 minute walk 10 oz water	Lunchtime: micronutrient-rich lunch 10 minute walk 10 oz water
Mid-day snack: Fruit! Nuts! Green Tea	Mid-day snack: Fruit! Nuts! Green Tea
PM: 15 minute household chores Dinner 15 minute walk after dinner Before Bed: 15 minute workout	PM: 15 minute household chores Dinner 15 minute walk after dinner Before Bed: 15 minute workout

Finding time to exercise daily is easy. Try this 15 minute exercise routine first thing in the morning to jumpstart your day!

Stretching (7 minutes)

Sit in a comfortable cross legged position on the floor.

- Neck rolls- rotate your head 3 times from right to left then 3 times for left to right
- Shoulder rolls- roll your shoulders forward and back 3 times in each direction
- Side stretches- place your left hand on the floor next to your hip, extend your right arm up, lend over to the left and stretch the right side of your body. Do the same to each side two times.

- Side twist- places your right hand on your left knee and your left hand on the floor behind your hip. Twist to the left. Do the same to each side two times.

Stretch your legs out while sitting on the floor.

- Leg lifts- place your hands down on either side your hips. Keeping your back straight, lift one leg at a time and hold it for 3 complete breaths. Repeat on each leg two times.

- Forward bends- lift both arms over head, take a deep breath, exhale and fold forward. Hold in the forward sitting position for 3 complete breaths.

Move to hand and knee position (Table Pose)

- Rolling hips- on hands and knees, roll your hips three times from right to left and then three times from left to right.

- Cat-Cow- on hands and knees, rotate your spine up and down by flexing and arching your back. Repeat 7 times.

Aerobics (5 minutes)

Standing

- Toe touches- stand with legs apart. Extend your arms sideways like the letter T. Inhale your breath. As you exhale, try to touch your right hand to your left foot. Inhale to standing. Exhale your left hand to your right foot. Repeat four times on each side.

- Jumping jacks- do jumping jacks for one minute. Build up each week until you can do them for 3 whole minutes!

- Jog or walk in place- whatever one you choose to do, be sure to lift your knees high and swing your arms. Jog or walk in place for one minute. Build up each week until you can move for 3 whole minutes!

Cool Down (3 minutes)

Lie down on the floor with knees bend and feet flat on the floor.

- Back massage- bring your knees into your chest and wrapping your arms around your legs. Rock side to side massaging your back.

- Hamstring release- Lie down on the floor with knees bend and feet flat on the floor. Extend right leg up towards the ceiling. Place your hands on the back of your thighs.

Inhale and lift your head towards your right knee. Hold for 2 breaths. Exhale and bring your head down. Repeat twice on each side.

- Reclining twist- bring your knees into your chest and wrapping your arms around your legs. Extend your arms sideways like the letter T, palms facing down on the floor. Inhale. Exhale and bring your legs over towards the right and turn your head towards the left. Repeat twice on each side.

- Reclining stretch- Lie on the floor with your arms extended. Stretch your body by flexing and pointing from your fingers to your toes, inhaling and exhaling as you stretch.

RESOURCE SECTION

FREQUENTLY ASKED QUESTIONS (FAQS)

The following are a list of the most common questions asked during the Healthy Weight, Healthy You! Workshop series. If you have any additional questions, please feel free to contact me at: Charlene@urbanherbalist.org or (443) 803-1179.

Q: What is the best artificial sweetener on the market today?

A: All artificial sweeteners provide the same benefit: empty calories with a sweet taste! Adding Splenda, Nutrisweet, or Sweet-n-Low isn't really supporting your goal of decreasing the amount of sugar carbs you eat. Also, there may be some health concerns associated with artificial (chemical) sweeteners as well. Most of the sugar carbs we eat are "hidden" because refined carbohydrates like French fries, potato chips, pasta and bread breakdown into simple sugars during digestion. This is the main source of weight gain. Is honey, agave nectar, maple syrup or brown sugar better than white sugar or sugar substitutes? In my opinion, no they are not. Local honey or raw honey does provide some additional sources of fiber and immune boosting qualities, however both local and raw sources of honey may be a challenge to come by and are expensive. Commercial honey is produced in ways that eliminates any real nutrient value from the product. Agave Nectar is like liquid jam, again some small benefit over white sugar or artificial sweeteners, but not that much. Brown sugar is basically white sugar with a little bit of molasses added to it. This includes raw sugar. Maple syrup that is 100% maple sap with no additives is the better choice.

If you really want a good source of sugar, black strap molasses would be my #1 choice. Not only is it sweet, it also contains a good source of potassium and iron. Yum!

Q: I am lactose intolerant and can't drink cow's milk. Is Soy or Almond Milk better for me?

A: Firstly, milk comes from mammals. Humans have their mother's milk as all other mammals do. We human though, have adjusted our palates to accept the taste of cow's milk and goat's milk- depending on how we are raised.

Nuts cannot produce "milk"- so Soy and Almond milk are artificial milk substitutes not milk.

I do not recommend these beverages because they contain lots of added sugar-especially the flavored brands of these products. There is also some controversy about the amount of soy products we have adopted into our diets and its impact on our endocrine system, with research showing soy constituents acting on estrogen receptors in our bodies. Elevated levels of estrogen have been linked to certain cancers.

In my opinion, milk is not a necessary requirement for our diet. Yes, milk products today are highly fortified with Vitamins A, D and calcium, however there are other natural sources for these vitamins and minerals in other whole foods, especially vegetables of the dark green leafy kind, and vegetables of the red, orange and yellow hue.

What do I use in my bowl of cereal or oatmeal? Try a cup of 100% apple juice. Yum!

Q: How much water should I drink everyday?

A: There are many opinions about the exact amount of water we need to drink daily. Some are: drink 1/3 of your body weight; drink 8-8 ounce glasses; drink an ounce of water for every pound that you weigh. Sounds like a lot of water and many trips to the potty!

We need to drink water to keep hydrated. Your skin, nails, eyes, sinuses and color of your urine are good indicators of how hydrated you are. I find, that the average person needs a minimum of 30 ounces of water daily. Water should be taken in throughout the day and not in one sitting (you will only eliminate it quickly!) Begin with 10 ounces first thing in the morning. Then pace the other 20 ounces throughout the day and don't drink anymore about one-hour or so before you go to bed or you will wake up during the night to relieve yourself.

If you drink caffeinated beverages like coffee or soda, then you'll need more water as caffeine acts as a diuretic. Drink a glass of water for every cup of coffee or can of soda you ingest.

Q: I don't like the taste of water. Can I drink flavored water instead?

A: No. H20 is Water. There is no real substitute. Flavored, sparkling and vitamin-induced "waters" are really juice-like beverages. Incidentally, juice does not constitute water and is not considered a water substitute either. You may get away with a non-caffeinated herbal tea that is not sweetened as a source of water. But pure H20 is best. If you need a little taste in your water, squeeze the juice of a <u>fresh</u> lemon or lime.

Q: Is it better for me to eat smaller meals more frequently throughout the day or stick to 3 meals: breakfast, lunch and dinner?

A: The best eating practice is to eat when you are hungry. The key is increasing your awareness so that you really understand that you are hungry and not simply responding to gastric clues from your tummy that has been habituated into eating at certain times of the day.

However, this will take some time.

If you have health challenges that include blood sugar balance, than your healthcare provider may have suggested that you eat smaller meals throughout the day. The challenge with this dietary strategy is portion sizing. What constitutes a "smaller meal?" To be successful in losing or maintaining your weight with this eating pattern requires that you plan out your meals carefully. You may try using *My Plate* (see Resources section) and designing three typical meals: breakfast, Lunch and dinner. Then divide each of the meals in half, and pace these 6 smaller meals throughout your day. You'll be getting the correct portions of the foods good for you to eat and staying within your optimal daily calorie intake range.

The three meals a day custom was established to support our traditional farming culture and the current food industry. Remember, food is fuel. You need an appropriate amount of food to fuel the activities of your day.

Q: I hate exercise! What can I do to motivate myself?

A: Motivation is a personal discipline that lives in your own heart and mind. We cannot buy it off the shelf. However, there are some simple ways to build your will to be more motivated. First, find an exercise and/or activity that you like to do. Just because you see the Striders run pasted your window every morning, doesn't mean this is the exercise for you. Walking, bowling, dancing, fishing, gardening, water aerobics, water jogging, hiking… there are many ways to get your body moving that is fun to do. Choose something easy that you like and set a time of day to practice and stick to it! Second, find a partner to exercise with. If your spouse, children or other family member doesn't want to join you, seek out someone else. Begin by joining a class or workshop and speak up about looking for an exercise group or partner. Partnerships are great motivators!

Q: Do I really need to take vitamin supplements? Can't I get all that I need from food?

A: As a practicing herbalist and nutritionist, I do recommend supplements based on the individual needs of a person. I also strongly believe that our current diet as well as the quality of the foods that are available does not provide the sufficient amount of nutrients we need for optimal health.

On the flip side, vitamin and herbal supplements have become big business and there is a lot of advertisement and other "infomercials" pushing these products. Be careful not to fall for the hype that either totes the curative benefits of certain supplements or that raises your panic level by leading you to believe you are deficient in certain ways.

The best approach to deciding if you need to take supplements and what kind is best for you to take, would be to begin with speaking to your healthcare provider. Inquired about your last set of blood work and see if there are any indications of vitamin or mineral deficiency. Why take more than you need? This could be more harmful than good.

If you like the idea of having a daily multi-vitamin, be sure that it is food-based supplement and not synthetic. Food-based supplements are more easily digested and "bio-available." How do I know what is a food-based? Read the label! A food-based multi-vitamin ingredient will list the actual food source for each vitamin and mineral included in the bottle. For example, if the supplement has Vitamin A, the source may be a food like "carrots."

Q: I know that vegetables are really good for you, but my family won't eat them. What can I do to encourage my family to eat healthier?

A: Most of us have not acquired a palate or taste for certain vegetables. We are use to the sweet and salty taste and basically reject any other flavor due to habit. The best way to encourage your family to eat healthier is to consistently offer healthier food choices. Try new recipes that will guide you on how to prepare the foods with herbs and spices that will enhance the flavor. Follow the recipe exactly as written until you begin to understand what herbs, spices and foods blend best together, then you can experiment. I've listed several recipes, cookbooks and on-line menu sources in the Resources Section of this workbook.

Q: I don't know how to shop for fresh produce. How can I tell if it's ripe or ready to eat?

A: The best quality vegetables and fruits are produced locally and in their season. Community Supported Agriculture groups or CSAs and local Farmers' Markets are great resources for learning about what foods are grown and produced locally and in season.

Grocery Stores get their produce from all over the world. This is the way we can have tomatoes and watermelon in December and January when they would not be in our own garden until late July – September. It is challenging to assess the ripeness and quality of fresh produce in grocery stores because foods come from long distances and probably have pesticides and other additives to support their transport and shelf life. The good news is that most grocery stores label the country and/or state of origin for their foods, so you can get a better perspective about where the food comes from. Meat products too! Most lamb is imported all the way from Australia!

A few tips may help you select the better quality of these foods: a gentle squeeze to feel for firmness (but not hard!); sniff for the fragrance of food- you should be able to smell its flavor. If it smells sour, not so good; check around for any bruising, brown spots or damage; and when in doubt asked the produce guy/gal!

Food staples to keep in your pantry

Keeping basic items in your pantry will ensure that you will always be prepared to cook a healthy and delicious meal. If you can't shop for them all right away, add one or two items to your shopping list each week. Be sure to restock them as you use them!

Canned Good
Canned fish (salmon or tuna)
Canned stewed tomatoes (NO SALT)
Canned whole cooked beans (NO SALT)
Condensed milk
Chicken broth (NO SALT)
Vegetable broth (NO SALT)
Canned Soups (LOW-SALT)
Tomato Paste

Grains
Long grain brown rice
Quick- cooking rolled oats
Whole wheat pastry flour
Whole wheat pasta
Whole Wheat Crackers
High Protein Cereal

Spices
Garlic powder
Turmeric
Onion powder
Ginger powder
Cayenne pepper
Oregano
Cinnamon
Thyme
Basil
Sea Salt
Baking Soda
Baking Powder
Brown Sugar
Olive Oil

Extras
Bottled Water
100% Fruit (Preserves or Jam)
Nut Butter (Almond or Peanut)
Dried Fruit (Raisins, cranberry, apricots)
Sunflower seeds
Whole Wheat Crackers
Honey

Frozen
Mixed vegetables
Mixed Fruit
Turkey Patties- Lean or low fat
Loaf of Whole Wheat Bread
Fish

How to shop on a low budget

You can save money and eat healthier too by changing how you shop and prepare for meals. Taking 30 minutes once and week to plan your menus will help you budget your groceries and ensure that you eat meals that are good and healthy for you.

Getting Started

1. Take a few minutes to make a weekly menu.
2. Make a list what you need to make each meal.
3. Look through your pantry and frig to see what stuff you already have and cross them off your list.
4. Look at sales flyers from your grocery store. Save money by planning meals based on what's on sale and what you already have in your kitchen.

While Shopping

1. Bring your list and coupons!
2. Buy food in quantities you will use before it goes bad.
3. Buy in bulk sale items that can be stored for a long time (and that you are sure to use!). If bulk items can be refrigerated or frozen, divide them into smaller portions and store them in freezer zip-lock bags.
4. Buy fruits and vegetables (produce) in season.
5. Take time to compare ingredients not just labels. Generic brand products usually have the same ingredients as brand name products and cost less.
6. Do not shop on an empty stomach. Shopping when you are hungry may cause you to buy things you don't need on impulse.

Where to Shop

Farmer's Markets: There's a lots of Farmers' Markets around! Many of the vendors take Food Stamps AND may double the value of your food stamps for shopping at the market.

Trader Joes: A whole sale grocery store that carries a good selection of organic foods at affordable prices. *http://www.traderjoes.com/*

Grocery Stores: Many grocery stores like Shoppers, Giant and Safeway carry organic foods. In fact both Giant and Safeway have their own organic food label. Giant (*Nature's Promise*) and Safeway (*Open Nature*) offers better quality foods for a few cents more than the usual brands. Look for these organic foods to go on sale and then stock up! Buy more and freeze them for later on in the month.

A week's worth of lunch menus for about $5/day

Make and take you lunch everyday can save you lots of money and help you stick to your weight loss goals. Create a weekly lunch menu that mixes and matches ingredients throughout the week. You only have to shop once!

Sunday	Spinach & Tomato Omelets 1-cup of strawberries 8 oz. of Ginger Green Tea
Monday	Humus Wrap Sandwich* Granny Smith Apple 1 cup of blue corn chips 8 oz. of Ginger Green Tea
Tuesday	Salmon salad over spinach 1 cup of blue corn chips 8 oz. of Ginger Green Tea
Wednesday	Green salad topped with cut-up cooked burger Cereal bar with fruit & seeds 8 oz. of Ginger Green Tea
Thursday	2 hardboiled eggs Blue corn chip salad* 8 oz. of Ginger Green Tea
Friday	Fish burritos (made with canned fish)* Mini veggie sticks with humus dip 8 oz. of Ginger Green Tea
Saturday	Ground turkey or beef burger topped with sauté spinach, onion and sunflower seeds Sliced apples and strawberries 8 oz. of Ginger Green Tea

Grocery List for Lunch Items: TOTAL COST $35.74
½ dozen eggs ($1.50) or carton of eggbeaters ($3.00)
Bag of spinach ($1.99)
2 Fresh tomatoes ($1.50)
Box of Ginger Green Tea ($2.99)
Canned Fish: Salmon ($3.00) or Tuna ($1.50)
3 Granny smith apples ($1.80)
Pint of strawberries ($2.99)
Humus ($2.50)
1 Onion ($0.69)
Bag of whole wheat tortillas ($2.50)

Box of frozen turkey or beef burgers ($.6.99)
Blue Corn Chips ($3.00)
Bag of carrots ($2.00)
Cucumber ($0.79)

*Quick Recipes

Humus Wrap Sandwich
Spread humus over whole wheat tortilla
Add veggies to taste: diced tomatoes, greens (spinach okay), cucumber, and 1 teaspoon of onions
Roll the tortilla
Wrap in plastic wrap

Fish Burritos
Open canned fish (Salmon or Tuna) and drain off water.
Add ½ of canned fish over whole wheat tortilla
Add veggies to taste: Add veggies to taste: diced tomatoes, greens (spinach okay), cucumber, and 1 teaspoon of onions
Roll the tortilla
Wrap in plastic wrap

Blue Corn Chip Salad
Is a disposable storage container, mix 1 cup of blue corn chips with diced tomatoes, cucumber, onions, greens, apples and sunflower seeds.
Top with 1 tablespoon of humus or any other salad dressing you like!

How to check Fast food menus and ingredients before going out

Fast food restaurant provide easy and inexpensive meals for busy families. But most fast foods are high in fats and calories that have little nutritional value.

Some fast-food restaurants are making changes to their menus in order to provide better quality food choices for their customers. These restaurants are also providing information about the ingredients in their menus so that you can make informed choices about what you eat.

Before you head out for take-out, take charge of your diet by looking at the ingredients in the restaurants menu. Most places have their menu information posted on-line so you can look at it and make meal decisions before you go.

Consider three critical facts when choosing menus:

1. ***Sugar, Sodium and Fat content***- large amount of these ingredients shows lots of calories that may satisfy you appetite and give you quick energy but not lots of nutrient value.

2. ***Portion Size***- this tells you how large the portion of food is or how many servings it contains.

3. ***Calories***- this tells you how many calories the portion of food contains. For example, if your goal is to eat 2000 calories per day, and you go to McDonald's and order a Double Quarter Pounder with Cheese (760 calories), large fries (500 calories) and the Chocolate McCaffe Shake (880 Calories), than you have eaten almost all of your daily calories in one meal.

Here are a few links to popular fast-food restaurants nutrition information page:

Subway
http://www.subway.com/applications/NutritionInfo/index.aspx

McDonald's
http://www.mcdonalds.com/us/en/food/food_quality/nutrition_choices.html

Panera Bread
http://www.panerabread.com/menu/

Wendy's
http://www.wendys.com/food/Nutrition.jsp

Week 1 Meal Planner

Day	Breakfast	Lunch	Dinner	Snack
Sunday	Scrambled Eggs, sautéed spinach, whole wheat toast w/ jam, 8 ounces water w/ squeeze of lemon	Sandwich with cheese, baby greens, cucumber and tomato slices, cup of corn chips, 100% fruit juice or herbal tea	Vegetarian Chili*, green salad, cup of brown rice, 8 ounces of water	1 cup of trail mix
Monday	1 1/2 cup of high protein cereal, 1 cup of low-fat milk, 1 piece of fresh fruit	2 cups of canned soup, toasted English muffin, herbal tea or sparkling water	Baked Fish, stemmed broccoli with red peppers & onions, cup of brown rice, 8 ounces of water	1 cup of fresh strawberries
Tuesday	bowl of fresh strawberries, one hard-boiled egg, 8 ounces of 100% fruit juice or herbal tea	leftover fish fillet sandwich with mixed greens and tomatoes on whole grain bread; cup of mixed fruit (grapes, melons), herbal tea or sparkling water	Bean and cheese Burritos (made with left over chili from Sunday evening), green salad, 8 ounces of water	2 cups of salt-free popcorn
Wednesday	1 1/2 cup of high protein cereal, 1 cup of low-fat milk, 1 piece of fresh fruit	Leftover bean and cheese burritos, granny smith apple, herbal tea or sparkling water	whole wheat pasta, sautéed ground turkey with carrots, onions and zucchini in low-sodium tomato sauce, 8 ounces of water	apple slices with peanut butter
Thursday	1 cup of low-fat yogurt with sliced bananas and 1/2 cup of granola; 100% fruit juice or herbal tea	veggie wrap: hummus, greens, cucumbers, tomatoes, onions; 100% fruit juice	baked fish fillets, sautéed veggies (zucchini, tomatoes, onions and green peppers); 1 cup of potato wedges, 8 ounces of water	blue corn chips and salsa
Friday	1 1/2 cup of high protein cereal, 1 cup of low-fat milk, 1 piece of fresh fruit	prepared vegetarian lasagna; sparkling water of herbal tea	Baked chicken, sautéed veggies (squash, carrots and onions), green salad, whole grain dinner roll, 8 ounces of water	2 oatmeal raisin cookies
Saturday	Fruit Smoothie*, whole wheat toast with butter.	whole grain toast with melted cheese and tomatoes; 1 cup of raw green beans and 3 tablespoons of low-fat salad dressing as a dip; herbal tea or sparkling water	Stirred-fry leftover chicken (chop in pieces); onions, carrots and broccoli; 1/4 cup of cooked brown rice all top over a bed of fresh spinach, 8 ounces of water	1 cup of frozen yogurt; 1/4 cup of nuts

Time Management for Cooking!

shop with a menu in mind
Look for coupons before you go to the grocery store
Cook main items on the weekend or when you have more time
Prep ahead of time by chopping fresh veggies and storing them in free
Make a little extra for leftovers!

Recipes of the Week!

Vegetarian Chili
Fruity Smoothie

Tips!

always carry your water bottle!
use your portion plate
carry your lunch to work or school

Week- 2 Meal Planner

Day	Breakfast	Lunch	Dinner	Snack
Sunday	Scrambled eggs with cheese and red peppers on English muffin; 8 ounces of cranberry juice	mixed fruit cup topped with 1/4 cup of yogurt and 2 tablespoons of high protein cereal (Like Great Grains or Kashi); 12 ounces water	Beef stew, green salad; 8 ounce of sparkling water	blue corn chips and salsa
Monday	Whole wheat toast with slice of cheese; piece of fresh fruit; 8 ounces of low fat milk	Leftover beef stew; 1 cup of green tea	2 cups of canned soup, salad, 1 slice of whole wheat toast and nut butter; 8 ounces of sparkling water	1 cup of Trail mix with assorted nuts and dark chocolate
Tuesday	Nut butter and jam whole wheat toast sandwich; piece of fresh fruit; 8 ounces of low-fat milk	Green salad, 1 cup of cooked broccoli with 1 slice of melted cheese; 1/2 whole wheat toast; 1 cup of green tea	baked chicken, green beans and baked red potato; 8 ounces of sparkling water	10 ounce bag of Kettle corn
Wednesday	1 & a half cups of high protein cereal (like Great Grains or Kashi); 1/2 of low-fat milk; piece of fresh fruit; 1 cup of green tea	leftover baked chicken, green salad; 8 ounces of 100% fruit juice	Baked fish with butter and lemon juice; 1 cup of brown rice; steamed broccoli (pour of a little of the fish butter & lemon sauce over it!); 8 ounces of sparkling water	2 oatmeal raisin cookies
Thursday	1 hard-boiled egg; 1 slice of toasted whole wheat toast with jam; 1 cup of green tea	Green salad topped with slices of left over fish and 2 tablespoons of brown rice; 1/2 whole grain roll; 8 ounces of 100% fruit juice	Sautéed vegetables (any mixed frozen vegetables will do!) served over brown rice; 1/2 grilled cheese sandwich; 8 ounces of sparkling water	5 ounces of frozen yogurt (in a cup rather than on a cone!)
Friday	1/2 grilled cheese sandwich; piece of fresh fruit; 1 cup of green tea	left over sautéed vegetables and rice; corn chips; 8 ounces of low-fat milk	home-made English muffin pizza with slice of cheese, 2 vegetable toppings of your choice; 8 ounces of sparking water	1 Breakfast bar
Saturday	8 ounces of yogurt with fresh fruit and 2 tablespoons of high protein cereal (like Great Grains or Kashi); 1 cup of green tea	left over home made pizza; 1 cup of 100% fruit juice	Turkey Pattie; green salad; 8 ounces of sparkling water	1 soft pretzel with no salt

Time Management for Cooking!

shop with a menu in mind
Look for coupons before you go to the grocery store
Cook main items on the weekend or when you have more time
Prep ahead of time by chopping fresh veggies and storing them in freezer bags for use during the week
Make a little extra for leftovers!

Recipe of the Week!

Beef Stew

Tips!

always carry your water bottle!
use your portion plate
carry your lunch to work or school

Shopping List for Weekly Menus

Here is a list of food supplies that will give you enough ingredients for two weeks of menus for a family of four. You can double the amount you buy and cook for leftovers throughout the week.

The items with a * can be bought either fresh or frozen.

Produce Section	Dairy Section	Meat Section	Frozen Foods	Aisle Section
2 bags of spinach	Eggs	Chicken	1 lb bag Mixed peppers*	Whole Wheat Bread
10 lb bag red potatoes	Low-fat milk	Ground Turkey*	1 lb bag Onions*	English Muffins
2 large onions*	Cheese		1 lb bag Mixed vegetables*	Nut butter- (peanut, almond, or sesame)
Fresh Vegetables*	Butter		1 lb bag Broccoli*	Fruit Jam or Jelly
Fresh Fruit*	Low-fat Yogurt		1 lb bag Mixed fruit	2 bottle of 100% Fruit juice*
3 lemons	Tortillas		2 lb bag of fish	Box of green tea
2 Tomatoes			Turkey Patties* (box of 12)	Canned Soup- low salt
1 cucumber				1 lb bag of Brown Rice
Bag of carrots				High Protein Cereal (like *Raisin Bran, Great Grains* or *Kashi*)
				Quick Oats
				15 oz Can of Fish (salmon or tuna)
				15 oz Can of Beans (black or red)
				Whole wheat pasta
				1 jar of tomato sauce- low salt
				Olive Oil
				Salad dressing- low fat
				Dried Fruit (like raisins or cranberries)
				Corn Chips

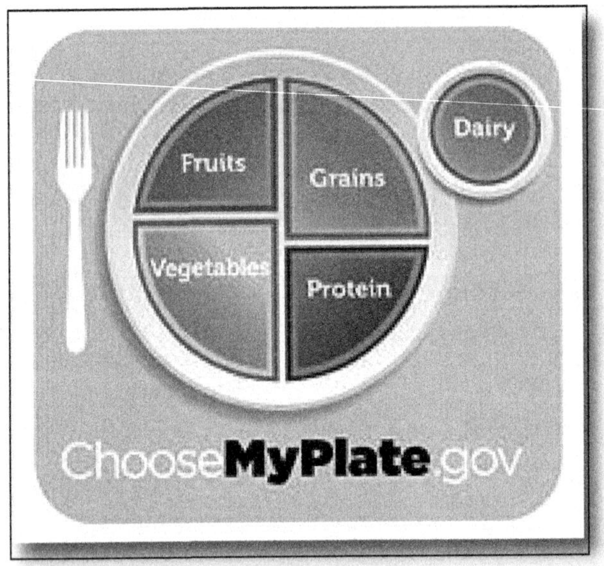
Fruits
Grains
Dairy
Vegetables
Protein
ChooseMyPlate.gov

Additional Resources By Section

I. Mind-Body Connection to Food

Nourishing Wisdom: a mind-body approach to nutrition and well-being. Author: Marc David. Bell Tower Press, 1991

When the body says no: understanding the stress-disease connection. Author: Gabor Mate, MD. John Wiley & Sons, Inc. 2003

Prakriti: your Ayurvedic constitution. Author: Dr. Robert E. Svoboda. Sadhana Publications, 1998

II. History of the American Diet

The Weight of the Nation (HBO Series) *www.theweightofthenation.hbo.com*

Ingredients: who's your farmer? (Pivot series) *www.ingredientsfilm.com/blog/?page_id=40*

Food, Inc. (movie) *www.takepart.com/foodinc*

III. Your Two Brains

Institute for the Psychology of Eating *http://psychologyofeating.com*

IV. Tools to increase our awareness for eating healthier

Digital App: WeightSnap. *WeightSnap* is a diet tracking cell phone App that helps you create a food diary by snapping photos of your meals to track and compare. The App allows you to keep notes about your meals, set goals and reminders and monitoring your weight loss progress by tracking your BMI and other physical weight loss indicators. *www.weightsnap.com*

V. What's the best diet on the market today?

READING FOOD LABELS
Center for Science in the Public Interest *www.cspinet.org*
Truth in Labeling *www.truthinlabeling.org*
International Food Information Council (IFIC) Foundation *www.foodinsight.org*
Food and Nutrition Information Center (USDA) *www.nal.usda.gov/fnic/*

VI. Simple steps for a healthier lifestyle

Staying Healthy with the Seasons. Author: Elson M. Haas, MD. Celestial Arts, 1981.

Encyclopedia of Natural Medicine: your comprehensive, user-friendly A-to-Z guide to treating more than 70 medical conditions- from arthritis to varicose veins, from cancer to heart disease. Authors: Michael Murray, ND; Joseph Pizzorno, ND. Prima Publishing, 1998.

Resolved: 13 Resolutions for Life. Author: Orrin Woodward. Obstacles Press, 2011.

VII. Kitchen Science Wisdom

Eat local and seasonal! Community Supported Agriculture. Local Harvest maintains a nationwide directory of small farms, farmers markets and other local food sources. *www.localharvest.org*

One Bite at a Time: Nourishing Recipes for Cancer Survivors and Their Friends. Authors: Rebecca Katz with Mat Edelson. Celestial Arts Press, 2004

Checkout Rebecca's website for more recipes: *www.rebeccakatz.com*

Food as Medicine: how to use diet, vitamins, juices, and herbs for a healthier, happier, and longer life. Author: Dharma Singh Khalsa, MD. Atria Books, 2003.

Healing with Whole Foods: Oriental Traditions and Modern Nutrition. Author: Paul Pitchford. North Atlantic Books, 1993.

Urban Pantry: tips & recipes for a thrifty, sustainable and seasonal kitchen. Author: Amy Pennington. Skiptone Press, 2010.

Nourishing Traditions: The Cookbook That Challenges Politically Correct Nutrition

and the Diet Dictocrats. Authors: Sally Fallon, Mary G. Enig, Ph.D. NewTrends Publishing, 1999.

The Moosewood Cook Book Series. Author: Mollie Katzen. Ten Speed Press.

Women, Food and God. Author: Geneen Roth.

A course in weight loss: 21 spiritual lessons for surrendering your weight forever. Author: Marianne Williamson.

VIII. Exercise, Mood and Food

Yoga Alliance Teacher/Studio Directory. *http://www.yogaalliance.org*

Fitnessglo: on-line exercise classes *http://www.fitnessglo.com/?gclid=CMqhkKmPg7wCFUjxOgodhSEA_w*

END NOTES

1. Chissell, M.D., John T. *Pyramids of power! An ancient African centered approach to optimal Health.* Positive Perceptions Publications. Baltimore, MD. 2000.
2. Wonder, Stevie. Higher Ground. *Innervisions* L.P. 1973
3. Chissell, page xxiv
4. Mills, Simon Y. *The essential book of herbal medicine.* Arkana Penguin Books. London. 1993. page 25
5. Bart, Lionel. Food. *Oliver! The Musical.* 1963.
6. The New College Edition of the American Heritage Dictionary of the English Language. Houghton Mifflin Company. Boston, MA. 1982.
7. Cordain, L. et al. *Origins and evolution of the Western diet: health implications for the 21st century*. American Journal of Clinical Nutrition 2005; 81:341-54.
8. Ibid
9. United States Department of Agriculture (USDA). *Healthy Eating Guidelines 2010*
10. Ibid
11. Cordain, L. et al.
12. Definition of Fat : MEDLINE PLUS
http://www.nlm.nih.gov/medlineplus/ency/article/002468.htm
13. Crayon, M.S., Robert. *Nutrition Made Simple: a comprehensive guide to the latest findings in optional nutrition.* M.Evans & Company. New York. 1994. Page 102.
14. USDA, pg 5
15. University of Maryland Medical Center. *Potassium.* http://www.umm.edu/altmed/articles/potassium-000320.htm
16. Imhoff, Daniel. *Food Fight: the citizen's guide to the next Food and Farm Bill. Watershed Media Book.* Healdsburg, CA. page 113
17. Imhoff, page 11
18. Definition of Couch Potato. Merriam Webster. http://www.merriam-webster.com/
19. Imhoff, page 186
20. Welsh, Susan O., and et al. USDA's *Food Guide: Background and Development.* Misc. Publication 1514. Nutrition Education Division, Human Nutrition Information Services, United States Department of Agriculture, Hyattsville, Md. September 1993, Page 1.

21. Ibid
22. Ibid
23. Ibid, page 3
24. Ibid, page 4-5
25. Imhoff, page 91
26. National Institutes of Health. *Relative intake of macronutrients impact of mild cognitive impairment or dementia and the Whitehall II Cohort Study*
Rhode Island Hospital: *A link between brain insulin resistance and neuronal stress in worsening Alzheimer's disease.*
27. *Insulin resistance in the brain: an old age or new age problem?* Biomedical Research Institute , University of Dundee, U.K.
28. http://medical-dictionary.thefreedictionary.com/Craving
29. Welsch, page 1
30. http://www.fda.gov/food/ingredientspackaginglabeling/labelingnutrition/ucm27.htm
31. Ibid
32. *http://www.fda.gov/food/ingredientspackaginglabeling/gras/ucm094040.htm*
33. Mayo Clinic. *Organic Foods: are they safer? More Nutritious?* http://www.mayoclinic.com/health/organic-food/NU00255
34. Patel, Raj. *Stuff and Starved: from farm to fork, the hidden battle for the world's food system.* Granta Books. London. 2008
35. Excerpt from: *http://www.allaboutwater.org/drink-water.html*
36. Feuerstein, George, Editor. *Yoga Gems: A treasury of practical and spiritual wisdom from ancient and modern masters.* Bantam Books, New York. 2002. Pg 100.
37 *The American Heritage Dictionary of the English Language*
38. Ibid
39. http://www.nutristrategy.com/index.htm

CPSIA information can be obtained
at www.ICGtesting.com
Printed in the USA
BVOW07s1313040917
493462BV00014B/35/P